MRCGP
Clinical Skills
Assessment:
Practice Cases

Third Edition

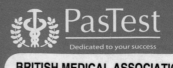

PasTest

Dedicated to your success

MRCGP
Clinical Skills
Assessment:
Practice Cases

Third Edition

Raj Thakkar
BSc (Hons) MBBS MRCGP MRCP (UK)
General Practitioner
Buckinghamshire

Edited by Meena Nathan

PasTest
Dedicated to your success

© 2014 PASTEST LTD
Egerton Court
Parkgate Estate
Knutsford
Cheshire
WA16 8DX

Telephone: 01565 752000

First Published 2009
Second Edition Published 2011
Third Edition Published 2014

ISBN: 9781905635894
           1905635893

A catalogue record for this book is available from the British Library.

The information contained within this book was obtained by the author from reliable sources. However, while every effort has been made to ensure its accuracy, no responsibility for loss, damage or injury occasioned to any person acting or refraining from action as a result of information contained herein can be accepted by the publishers or author.

All references valid at time of publication.

PasTest Revision Books and Intensive Courses

PasTest has been established in the field of undergraduate and postgraduate medical education since 1972, providing revision books and intensive study courses for doctors preparing for their professional examinations.

Books, courses and online revision available for:

Medical undergraduates, MRCGP, MRCP Parts 1 and 2, MRCS, MRCPCH Parts 1 and 2, DCH, MRCOG, DRCOG, FRCA, Dentistry.

For further details contact:

PasTest, Freepost, Knutsford, Cheshire WA16 7BR

Tel: 01565 752000   Fax: 01565 650264

www.pastest.co.uk   enquiries@pastest.co.uk

Text prepared in the UK by Carnegie Book Production, Lancaster

Printed and bound in the UK by Page Bros Ltd, Norwich

CONTENTS

ACKNOWLEDGEMENTS

I would like to acknowledge, with thanks, the following for their contribution to this book, and for permission kindly granted:

Meena Nathan

Alice Barnes

Peter Havelock

Duncan Rourke

British Heart Foundation

British Hypertension Society

British Thoracic Society

GMC

Meningitis.org

MIMS

NICE

Raj Thakkar would also like to acknowledge Lily Atkins for her hard work.

To my wonderful family, for many untold reasons.

ABOUT THE AUTHOR

Raj Thakkar BSc (Hons) MBBS MRCGP MRCP (UK) gained his neuroscience and medical degrees from University College London. During his vocational training in the Oxford Deanery, he won the national GP enterprise award, registrar division. He currently works as a GP partner and commissioning director in Buckinghamshire, where his special interests include cardiovascular medicine. He is an award winning author and works as a freelance writer, as well as appearing regularly on the radio.

ABOUT THE CONTRIBUTORS

Meena Nathan BSc (Hons) BM DFFP MRCGP Derm Dip (PG) gained her biomedical sciences and medical degree at the University of Southampton. She completed her vocational training in the Oxford Deanery. Currently working as a GP partner in Hertfordshire, her special interests include women's health, family planning and dermatology.

Peter Havelock MBBS, FRCGP graduated from St Mary's London in 1970 and became a general practitioner in Wooburn Green, Buckinghamshire. He has been involved in teaching for many years, being a trainer, course organiser, RCGP examiner and Associate Director in the Oxford Deanery. His special interests within teaching have been teaching and learning around the doctor/patient consultation. He has been the author of many papers and books about the subject and has run courses for hundreds of trainers and registrars around the UK. He has recently retired from general practice.

INTRODUCTION

This book aims to prepare the candidate efficiently for the CSA (clinical skills assessment) element of the MRCGP. It follows extensive questioning of candidates, past and present, about what they want from a CSA preparation book. The resulting book has, at its core, four 'exam circuits' that simulate the CSA experience as closely as possible.

A bonus case has been included at the end of each examination circuit. These cases are merely designed to add richness to the book, reflect the type of cases that you would expect in everyday general practice, and hence what you may experience in the CSA.

All the cases in this book are set out with the intention that candidates can role-play consultations and maximise their learning from each scenario. I try to provide the 'candidate' and the 'actor' with information as it would be presented in the exam. Along with the notes for the candidate, each case has a blank page on which candidates are encouraged to 'brainstorm' and gather their thoughts prior to each case. You are encouraged to try to anticipate what might be expected from the case, to allow subsequent reflection on how these 2 minutes are best spent for you in the real exam.

A commentary is then provided on the intended learning points with reference to the CSA marking schedule, as well as key learning points and references. Each case in this book has been designed to bring out particular skills and behaviours required for the CSA and hence independent practice. Each 'exam' has been constructed to reflect the spread of curriculum domains that you may see in the real exam, and to cover the different types of consultation with their differing agendas and primary aims, which again can be anticipated in the real exam. A table is provided at the start of each circuit, showing the case mix for each mock exam.

To pass the CSA a candidate must demonstrate a patient-centred approach to gathering information, an ability to assess and process this information and to construct evidence-based management plans. The consultation should flow, keeping the patient on-board and demonstrating insight into his or her thought process. To meet these standards, I try to present information in a way that assists the development of a methodical approach to consulting, with particular acknowledgement of the CSA requirements.

To address the nuts and bolts of the exam, I have incorporated introductory sections that cover frequently asked questions, tips for success, with personal experience from recently successful candidates. To address the history of the exam and the finer points of consultation techniques I include a commentary by Peter Havelock, co-author of the acclaimed texts, *The Consultation* and *The New Consultation* (see below)

To make the most of this book, I recommend that cases be practised under examination conditions with a strict adherence to time-keeping. You may want to practise a whole examination all at once or, alternatively, discuss each case after you have role-played, teasing out the various issues and then role-playing again using different consultation styles and techniques, until you have found one that works for you. I envisage the book being used in small groups of GP 'registrars', although it might appeal to the lone learner as well. Of course, this book cannot be an exhaustive coverage of all the cases that could present themselves in the CSA exam, although I hope that it encourages the reflective stepwise approach that will safeguard, as far as possible, against failure.

Revision does not stop with this book and every case that you see in your daily practice should be considered a CSA case. After all, the MRCGP is designed not to test your knowledge of esoteric medicine, but to reflect everyday, high-quality general practice.

REFERENCES

Pendleton D, Schofield T, Tate P, Havelock P. *The Consultation: An approach to teaching and learning*. Oxford: Oxford University Press, 1984.

Pendleton D, Schofield T, Tate P, Havelock P. *The New Consultation*. Oxford: Oxford University Press, 2003.

ABBREVIATIONS

ACE	angiotensin-converting enzyme
ACEI	ACE inhibitor
ACR	albumin : creatinine ratio
A&E	accident and emergency department
AF	atrial fibrillation
AKT	applied knowledge test
AV	atrioventricular node
AVRT	atrioventricular re-entry tachycardia
BM	blood glucose
BMI	body mass index
BNF	*British National Formulary*
BP	blood pressure
BTS	British Thoracic Society
CbD	case-based discussion
CBT	cognitive behavioural therapy
CCF	congestive cardiac failure
CCG	clinical commissioning group
CCT	certificate of completion of training
CEO	chief executive officer
CFC	chlorofluorocarbon
CLL	chronic lymphoblastic leukaemia
COPD	chronic obstructive pulmonary disease
COT	consultant observation tool
CRP	C-reactive protein
CRT	capillary refill time
CSA	clinical skills assessment
CVD	cardiovascular disease
CXR	chest radiograph
DEXA	dual-energy X-ray absorptiometry
DVT	deep vein thrombosis
ECG	electrocardiogram
EER	experimental event rate

eGFR	estimated glomerular filtration rate
ESR	erythrocyte sedimentation rate
FBC	full blood count
FEV_1	forced expiratory volume in 1 second
FP10	blank prescription
FVC	forced vital capacity
GFR	glomerular filtration rate
GI	glycaemic index
GMC	General Medical Council
GMS	General Medical Services
HAD	hospital anxiety and depression score
Hb	haemoglobin
HCA	health care assistant
hCG	human chorionic gonadotrophin
HDL	high-density lipoprotein
HR	heart rate
HRT	hormone replacement therapy
ICD	internal cardioverter–defibrillator
ICS	inhaled corticosteroid
JVP	jugular venous pressure
LABA	long-lasting β antagonist
LAT	local area team
LVF	left ventricular failure
MA	meta-analysis
MAOI	monoamine oxidase inhibitor
MCH	mean corpuscular haemoglobin
MCV	mean corpuscular volume
MI	myocardial infarction
MMR	measles, mumps and rubella
MRC	Medical Research Council
MRI	magnetic resonance imaging
MRSA	meticillin-resistant *Staphylococcus aureus*
MSF	multi-source feedback
MSU	midstream urine
NAD	no abnormalities detected

NICE	National Institute for Health and Care Excellence
NNT	number needed to treat
nocte	every night
NTA	National Treatment Agency
NSAID	non-steroidal anti-inflammatory drug
NSTEMI	non-ST-elevation myocardial infarction
OA	osteoarthritis
OCD	obsessive–compulsive disorder
od	*omni die* (once daily)
o/e	on examination
PCL	posterior cruciate ligament
PCT	primary care trust
PCOS	polycystic ovary syndrome
PCR	polymerase chain reaction
PE	pulmonary embolus
PEFR	peak expiratory flow rate
PHQ-9	patient health questionnaire
PID	pelvic inflammatory disease
PMB	postmenopausal bleeding
PMETB	Postgraduate Medical Education and Training Board
PMR	polymyalgia rheumatica
POP	progestogen-only pill
PR	per rectum
prn	as required
PSA	prostate-specific antigen
PT	prothrombin time
PUVA	psoralens + UVA
QALY	quality-adjusted life-year
qds	*quarter die sumendum* (to be taken four times a day)
QOF	Quality and Outcomes Framework
RCGP	Royal College of General Practitioners
RCT	randomised controlled trial
RICE	rest, ice, compression and elevation
RR	respiratory rate
RRR	relative risk reduction

RSV	respiratory syncytial virus
SCC	squamous-cell carcinoma
SD	standard deviation
SIGN	Scottish Intercollegiate Guidelines Network
SLE	systemic lupus erythematosus
SLS	selected list scheme
βhCG	β-human chorionic gonadotrophin
SMART	Sameterol Muticentre Asthma Research Trial
SOB	shortness of breath
SSRI	selective serotonin reuptake inhibitor
STEMI	ST-elevation myocardial infarction
STI	sexually transmitted infection
T_3	triiodothyronine
T_4	thyroxine
TB	tuberculosis
tds	*ter die sumendum* (to be taken three times a day)
TED	thromboembolic deterrent
TENS	transcutaneous electrical stimulation
TFT	thyroid function test
THR	total hip replacement
TIA	transient ischaemic attack
TSH	thyroid-stimulating hormone
2WW	two week wait
U&Es	urea and electrolytes
UTI	urinary tract infection
URTI	upper respiratory tract infection
UVA	long-wavelength ultraviolet (light)
VEGF	vascular endothelial growth factor
WCC	white cell count
WPBA	workplace-based assessment
WPW	Wolff–Parkinson–White Syndrome
WOMAC	Western Ontario and McMaster Universities Index of Osteoarthritis

Chapter 1
FAQs and tips
for success

If you let it, the CSA can hover over your GP registrar year like a black cloud. It doesn't need to. The RCGP has spent time and energy perfecting this examination to make sure that it does exactly what it says on the tin. It assesses you 'doing the day job', just as it should. So, if you structure your registrar year using all possible resources and prepare properly for both the AKT and the CSA, there should be no surprises when it comes to the day of the assessment.

Here are some 'top tips' of how to succeed in the CSA.

BEFORE THE DAY

Tip

    ✓   **DON'T NEGLECT BASIC CLINICAL KNOWLEDGE**

Don't make the mistake of assuming that the CSA is purely a test of your communication skills. Focus your revision on topics that you find difficult or those that you're least experienced in. After each surgery keep a logbook of cases or topics you found difficult and why (DEN = doctor educational need). Read up on the clinical aspects **the same day** if at all possible, or discuss them with your trainer at your debrief.

Tip

    ✓   **DON'T PREPARE FOR THE CSA IN ISOLATION**

It is difficult to 'revise' for these examinations in the way that you may have done for other more traditional written assessments. Preparation for the CSA should be an ongoing project and an integral part of daily life as a GP trainee. Don't underestimate how valuable videoing your consultations can be.

WHAT TO WEAR

- Smart clothes that would be appropriate if you were working as a locum GP in a new practice
- This does not have to mean tie and suit for men, although a pair of polished shoes go a long way
- Avoid wearing anything too risqué (men and women).

FORMAT OF EXAM

- Simulated surgery of 13 cases (previously this included a dummy case; however, all will be scored as of September 2010)

- An iPad with an RCGP app containing a list of the patients whom you will see during your assessment. Full information is available on the RCGP website

- 10 minutes each case

- 2 minutes between patients to read the notes for the following case; make the most of this time

Tip

   ✓ **Read each case one at a time so that you can focus on the case in hand.**

CASE MIX IN EXAM

- Thought is given to the spread of cases in each exam, so that as many domains and clinical systems are covered while testing as many varied skills as possible.

- See the domain coverage grids appended to each of the four exam circuits in this book.

- You can expect a fairly even mix of age and gender, of acute, chronic and health promotion, and of clinical systems.

- There will be a mix of 'primary aims' being tested among the cases within each exam circuit, eg acute and ongoing medical management, practical skills, health promotion, psychosocial issues, diversity issues, ethical issues, handling anger, low mood, anxiety and demanding patients.

- Expect at least one home visit or telephone consultation.

WHY PEOPLE FAIL

- Poorly structured consultation

- Did not develop appropriate management plan (usually because ran out of time – take a watch or clock)

- Did not recognise the challenge (failure avoided if pick up on cues, allow the patient to talk with open questions, and ensure that ideas, concerns and expectations [ICE] are covered)

- Did not develop a shared management plan (failure avoided if the patient is presented with 'options', and if understanding of ongoing management including follow-up and safety netting is checked).

WHERE IS THE EXAM HELD?

- Visit the RCGP website for full information on the venue and a virtual tour for those who want to get the adrenaline really pumping.

Tip

   ✓ **Book a hotel/B&B nearby the night before to avoid the added stress of commuting to the exam from distance. If you consider that your exam fee will be forfeited if you do not arrive for the exam on time, the extra cost of a hotel room can be viewed as a wise insurance policy.**

WHAT DO YOU NEED TO TAKE TO THE EXAM?

- See RCGP website for the list

- Don't forget your photo ID.

Tip

   ✓ **Fold pages or insert 'sticky tabs' in your BNF (which should not be written in) to give you the confidence of finding specific sections more quickly.**

MARKING SCHEME

- Marks are awarded in three broad areas for each case: data gathering, clinical management and interpersonal skills

- Descriptors of what skills are being assessed in these areas can be viewed at www.rcgp.org.uk. There are four possible overall marks for each of the 13 cases: clear pass, pass, fail and clear fail

- Descriptors for these marks can be viewed at www.rcgp-curriculum.org.uk

- There is a 'borderline averaging' system to ensure that people are not unfairly marked down if a specific circuit is harder than the next.

WHEN IS THE CSA EXAM?

- See dates on RCGP website

Tip

- ✓ **Do not miss the application deadlines**

WHEN SHOULD YOU SIT THE CSA EXAM?

- 'When you are ready'

- For most people this is after they have passed the AKT, and usually some time in the final registrar year

- Given the expense entailed, this is an exam that you do not want to fail and so there is an argument for gaining as much experience as possible before making an attempt

- The flipside to this approach is that if you fail the exam late in your registrar year you may be forced to add a further 6 months to your training

- Your trainer is usually best placed to assist you in this sometimes difficult decision.

WHAT CLINICAL EXAMINATIONS MIGHT BE EXPECTED?

- Common sense really, and worth some forethought

- Consider how you might ask permission to examine different body parts and systems being polite and using lay language, eg NOT 'cranial nerves', but perhaps 'nerves in your head'

- Think about how you might perform examinations from a problem-based approach (eg 'short of breath') as opposed to the hospital medicine systems approach (eg cardiovascular or respiratory systems)

- Discuss this with your trainer to ensure that all the bases are covered – this makes for a good tutorial.

Tip

✓ It is a good time to go back to basics. And dust off your medical school textbooks. Discipline yourself to do proper examinations in your consultations, as if it were the real thing. GP examinations need to be targeted and focused. It might be useful to write down a pro forma for each examination to help you to think things through logically.

CHAPTER 1

CHAPTER 1

DURING THE EXAM

- Forget the previous case and focus on reading the notes for the next case in the 2 minutes allowed

- Introduce yourself, check the name of the patient/person attending the consultation, and offer/help them to a seat

- Close the door behind the patient

- 'What has brought you in today?' = open question that allows actor to give the 'opening line'

- 'Please tell me a bit more about that?' = second open question allows actor to give information 'freely divulged in response to open questions'

- Verbally comment on any verbal or non-verbal clues to demonstrate your patient-centredness and your active listening, and to help uncover any hidden agendas (eg 'You look troubled by that ... that must be difficult ... .') – without being cheesy and unnatural!

- Ask ICE questions = 'What do you think might have caused this? Do you have any worries about this? What were you hoping we would be able to do about this today?' Remember to cover red flags and ask specific questions to hone in on the diagnosis.

- Ask psychosocial questions = 'How is this impacting on your life? What are your home circumstances? Why now?'

- Summarise back to the patient to show that you have listened, to uncover any information missed first time around, and to check your understanding of why they have attended referencing their ideas, concerns, and expectations

- Have you understood the patient and has the patient understood you?

- Offer to examine if appropriate, asking permission and briefly outlining what you would like to examine in lay language and why

- Avoid causing discomfort by asking if the patient has any pain anywhere

- Explain what you are doing as you go along using lay language

- Summarise your findings and explain what you think the problem might be and what it might not be with reference to patient's ICE

- Provide the patient with management options that adhere to evidence-based medicine, unless you identify an emergency where options might not be appropriate

- 'Hand over' to the patient, allowing him or her to choose the preferred management plan

- Summarise plan and check understanding: 'Is there anything I have said that you did not understand?'

- Check that you have a shared understanding of management plan and outline safety nets to cover different eventualities as appropriate.

Tip

✓ **FIND CONSULTATION MODELS THAT SUIT YOU, AND PRACTISE THEM**

Early in the registrar year, learn about the different consultation models and think about what works best for you. It's OK to dip into a number of different models and piece together your preferred approach. Be strict with yourself, and set yourself challenges in each surgery (or at least each time that you video) to work on a particular area of your consultation style. For instance, in one surgery you could focus on different ways of negotiating shared management plans with patients. Before the CSA, each surgery should be treated like an examination. If you do this, by the time the CSA comes around, your consultations will be well structured and patient centred.

Tip

✓ **PUT UP A CRIB SHEET IN YOUR CONSULTING ROOM**

This should detail the structure of your 'perfect' consultation with your favoured phrases highlighted so that you can become practised in using them. Patient-centred consulting styles will become second nature by the time you sit the CSA.

Tip

✓ **USE YOUR TRAINER**

Joint surgeries and use of the eportfolio, COTs, video assessments and role-play are great ways for your trainer to see how you are doing, and for you to practise what you've learnt in front of an expert. Although this may feel daunting, you will really benefit from the input. Another benefit of joint surgeries is that you get used to having a third person in the consultation, as there will be in the CSA. It puts you on the spot in a different way and makes you put some of the techniques that you've read about into practice.

HOW TO CONSULT IN 10 MINUTES

- You are not expected to write clinical notes in the CSA, which probably gives you an extra 1–2 minutes than you have in reality.

- CSA cases are fair in that they are achievable in 10 minutes, unlike some cases in the real world which can require a lot longer.

- Discuss time management with your trainer.

- Sit in with colleagues to see how they do it.

Tip

✓ **Ensure that you have all the structural elements of a 'perfect' consultation in place before you start worrying about reducing your consultation time during your registrar year. Better to get the engine tuned before you start trying to move through the gears!**

WHAT HAPPENS ON THE DAY?

- You have to arrive at least an hour before the start of the exam and are briefly quarantined in a room if you are sitting the exam in the afternoon, to avoid any contact with the morning's candidates who will process out of the building before you are allowed to emerge.

- There is a short briefing.

- Your equipment has to be in a clear plastic bag (provided) with other belongings placed in your locker.

- After the briefing you will be shown to your 'consulting room' and given a few minutes to settle in. On the desk you'll find pencils and all manner of forms (blood/X-ray forms, peak expiratory flow (PEFR) charts, prescription pads and medical certificates); a clock is in easy view. Then there are the case notes, on an iPad. It is held in a frame. When you enter the room the iPad is ready for you to log in using your GMC number.

Please refer to the RCGP website for further information.

- An odd sounding buzzer will ring, and the first patient will knock on the door and be followed in by the examiner.

- You should ignore the examiner who will try to sit out of your line of sight as much as possible. Be nice to the patients/actors, just as you normally would be with a patient. Be polite and courteous, introduce yourself and then get going.

- Time is an issue, so just do your best. If a patient comes in with deep, difficult issues, go with it. Don't try to rush things to tick all the boxes. Just make the best possible use of time. On the other hand, don't draw things out unnecessarily. If the case seems straightforward and you finish early that's fine. Just run through your checklist structure, and then end the consultation. By finishing just a little early it gives you a longer break between patients – a much-needed breather.

- You may be required to examine any system on the day. If you feel that an intimate examination would be appropriate, offer this to the examiner and patient in the CSA. Say something like, 'Normally I would proceed to do a rectal examination'. Clearly they will stop you, but at least they know that you are thinking about it. Don't be thrown if you are offered a manikin to examine, however. Think about how you'd approach that kind of situation in a CSA station.

- Use the 2 minutes between patients to put all that has happened behind you, and read the next set of case notes.

- Halfway through the examination, you will be ushered out of your room for a coffee and toilet break. (You will find that even trips to the toilet have to be accompanied by an invigilator.) You are not allowed to discuss cases with the other candidates as you will all see them at different times and so might inadvertently forewarn/mislead/scare!

- During your preparations think about how you'd handle the following consultations in the CSA:

  - telephone consultations

  - consultations with a member of staff about a patient or colleague problem

CHAPTER 1

- consultations with family members about patients (a great way to test your understanding of confidentiality and/or consent)

- consultation with a deaf/blind person

• consultation with a patient with learning difficulties and the carer

• paediatric consultations (with either parents or young adolescents).

Tip

✓ **Be yourself and try to treat the CSA as if it were normal surgery. Make sure that you have plans to celebrate when it's all over. You will deserve a pat on the back.**

USEFUL RESOURCES

- Websites: RCGP, PastTest cases online, GPonline.com, several GP trainee websites from around the country as sources of further written cases and tips

- Books: google 'MRCGP CSA' and see Amazon site for range of CSA books

- DVDs: GPonline.com (*Effective Consulting* with Peter Tate, co-author of *The New Consultation*), RCGP, Wessex Deanery; several other GP trainee websites from around the country give further details on this

- Colleagues: fellow trainees, trainers, course organisers

- Thakkar, R. *MIMS Consultation Guide*, Haymarket Publishing, 2012.

Chapter 2
The CSA examination: history and overview

'An assessment of the doctor's ability to integrate and apply appropriate clinical, professional, communication and practical skills in general practice.'

Definition of the purpose of the CSA

RCGP

The CSA examination is a clinical consulting skills examination, based on cases from general practice, with the role players as patients and experienced MRCGP assessors. The assessment is able to provide a pre-determined, standardised level of challenge to the candidates. It is derived from the video component and the simulated surgery of the previous MRCGP. The advantage of the CSA as an assessment process is that it assesses the clinical skills of the candidates in a wide range of situations. The CSA triangulates information from the other aspects of the MRCGP: the workplace-based assessment and the applied knowledge test. The use of simulated patients is a well-tried technique, and is valid for testing clinical skills. It is essential that the case production is quality assured and the role players and the assessors are well trained and monitored. The CSA is based on the Royal College of General Practitioners' (RCGP's) curriculum, and the cases are selected to include the wide spectrum found in everyday general practice. The RCGP website describes the CSA and points out those areas of the curriculum that are particularly tested.

The CSA tests mainly from the following areas of the curriculum:

Primary care management – recognition and management of common medical conditions in primary care.

Problem-solving skills – gathering and using data for clinical judgement, choice of examination, investigations and their interpretation. Demonstration of a structured and flexible approach to decision-making.

Comprehensive approach – demonstration of proficiency in the management of co-morbidity and risk.

Person-centred care – communication with patient and the use of recognised consultation techniques to promote a shared approach to managing problems.

Attitudinal aspects – practising ethically with respect for equality and diversity, with accepted professional codes of conduct.

The CSA will also test:

Clinical practical skills – demonstrating proficiency in performing physical examinations and using diagnostic/therapeutic instruments.

The role players are professionally trained and will play the same role about 28 times in a day. Their roles are written to enable them to respond to the appropriate questions and communication skills from the candidate. They need to be treated with respect and courtesy and the examination needs to be done carefully and with empathy; they have no assessment role. The assessors are unobtrusive and their only task is to mark the candidates.

THE MECHANISMS OF THE CSA

The candidates will all be tested at the same purpose-modified test centre, currently in Euston. The CSA is run a number of times a year (see www. rcgp.org.uk), and candidates may apply any time within the ST3 year and take it more than once (see Chapter 1). The format is: 13 simulated patient consultations; each patient is accompanied by an assessor who will remain with the same case each time. There is an initial briefing and you will be shown to your room. In the room will be an iPad with the case notes for each patient in order, blank prescriptions (FP10) and blank certificates (fit notes; the new Med 3). The role players and assessors will be shown to your room; the cases last 10 minutes with a 2 minute break between cases. A buzzer will sound to mark the start and the end of the cases; there will be a 15-minute break after the seventh case with an opportunity to go to the toilet and have refreshments. A clinical examination may be required, but the patient may decline to be examined; there are no intimate examinations. Which clinical examination you choose, and how you perform will be marked. There might be important physical signs.

You can write on the notes provided, but they have no part in the marking and are not to be removed from the room. The prescriptions or certificates are to be given to the role player, and they may be marked.

THE MARKING SCHEDULE

Each case is marked in three domains:

1. Data-gathering, technical and assessment skills

2. Clinical management skills

3. Interpersonal skills.

DATA-GATHERING, TECHNICAL AND ASSESSMENT SKILLS

Gathering and using data for clinical judgement, choice of examination, investigations and their interpretation. Demonstrating proficiency in performing physical examinations, and using diagnostic and therapeutic instruments.

CLINICAL MANAGEMENT SKILLS

The recognition and management of common medical conditions in primary care. Demonstrating a structured and flexible approach to decision-making. Demonstrating the ability to deal with multiple complaints and co-morbidity. Demonstrating the ability to promote a positive approach to health.

INTERPERSONAL SKILLS

Demonstrating the use of recognised communication techniques to understand the patient's illness experience and develop a shared approach to managing problems. Practising ethically with respect for equality and diversity, in line with the accepted codes of professional conduct.

All three domains have equal weighting and assessors use word pictures to help them decide which grade to give for each domain, and then use this information to make a judgement on the case overall. On the marking schedule there is a box for serious concerns that, fortunately, is used only rarely. The assessor will also make notes for feedback to the candidates.

CHAPTER 2

Chapter 3
Consultation skills in the CSA

The clinical skills assessment (CSA), as the name indicates, is focused on the work that the GPs do in their consulting rooms with patients. This was very well described nearly 50 years ago by Sir James Spence and it is the candidate's competency at this that the CSA strives to assess.

> 'The essential unit of medical practice is the occasion when, in the intimacy of the consulting room or sick room, a person who is ill or believes himself to be ill, seeks the advice of a doctor whom he trusts. This is a consultation and all else in the practice of medicine derives from it. The purpose of the consultation is that the doctor, having gathered his evidence, shall give explanation and advice.'
>
> Spence[1]

As the box above suggests, the consultation is the cornerstone of general practice. The average GP registrar will have more than 4000 consultations in 12 months, and if they continue a career in general practice will conduct more than 100 000 face-to-face consultations. It is not surprising that the MRCGP has a very strong focus on the consultation and therefore in the teaching; over the ST3 year the consultation is constantly discussed and assessed. The CSA should not be looked at in isolation because many of the areas of the curriculum covered in the CSA are also covered in the workplace-based assessment. Clearly the consultant observation tool (COT) is focused on the consultation; the feedback in these sessions is essential in developing the registrar's skills in the consultation. It is thus important to do many more COT assessments than the minimal. The COT assessment criteria give the registrars clear guidance on the elements of 'an effective consultation'.

CHAPTER 3

- Encourage the patient's contribution

- Respond to cues

- Place complaint in appropriate psychosocial contexts

- Explore patient's health understanding

- Include or exclude likely relevant significant condition

- Make an appropriate physical or mental state examination

- Make an appropriate working diagnosis

- Explain the problem in appropriate language

- Seek to confirm that the patient understands

- Make an appropriate management plan

- Give the patient the opportunity to be involved in significant management decisions

- Make effective use of resources

- Specify conditions and interval for follow-up

The COT assessment criteria

The sensible registrar will work at each of the criteria to understand the evidence for it, to master the strategies and skills that are needed to achieve it, and to practise their skills in their day-to-day consultations.

THE RELATIONSHIP OF THE CSA TO THE RCGP CURRICULUM

Over the last few years there has been a great deal of work within the RCGP to create and coordinate the GP curriculum with the end point assessment of GP training. This has been stimulated by the Postgraduate Medical Education and Training Board (PMETB) which has set standards for the training of doctors. Information and an explanation of the work of this important organisation can be found on their website, www.pmetb.org.uk where the start of the page 'about us' is:

'PMETB is the independent regulatory body responsible for postgraduate medical education and training. We ensure that postgraduate training for doctors is of the highest standard.' Their remit covers all the Royal Colleges.

The GP Curriculum should be well known to all trainee doctors considering a career in general practice and is found on the RCGP website, www.rcgp-curriculum.org.uk. There are specific areas of the curriculum that are particularly assessed by the CSA and some of the domains more obviously covering the whole area of consultation skills are:

• **Primary care management** – recognition and management of common medical conditions in primary care.

• **Problem-solving skills** – gathering and using data for clinical judgement, choice of examination, investigations and their interpretation, and the demonstration of a structured and flexible approach to decision-making.

• **Comprehensive approach** – demonstration of proficiency in the management of co-morbidity and risk.

• **Person-centred care** – communication with patient and the use of recognised consultation techniques to promote a shared approach to managing problems.

• **Attitudinal aspects** – practising ethically with respect for equality and diversity, with accepted professional codes of conduct.

• **Clinical practical skills** – demonstrating proficiency in performing physical examination and using diagnostic/therapeutic instruments.

In this chapter I will not be going into the detail of these aspects of the curriculum, but it is essential that candidates are aware of them early in their training and have realised what knowledge and skills they need to learn and what attitudes are important in helping a consultation be effective. It is obvious that people learn best when they are clear what it is that they have to learn; GP trainees need to be clear about the GP curriculum and use it daily to drive their learning.

CHAPTER 3

HOW TO USE ALL YOUR ST3 YEAR TO DO WELL IN THE CSA CONSULTATION SKILLS

In the last paragraph I suggested that the GP registrar should be steeped in the RCGP curriculum, but I recognise that it can be seen as a mammoth task. Do not be put off but take it in bite-size pieces. The place to start is in the first two sections of the core and extended statements of the curriculum documents (www.rcgp-curriculum.org.uk) They are:

- Being a GP

- The general practice consultation.

These will give the trainee a clear idea on what to learn. How to learn is a different matter and the Curriculum guide for Learners and Teachers from the RCGP is a very good start. It is recognised that different learners have different preferences on how they learn, but it is clear that they learn best when different learning methods or modalities are combined, eg by seeing, listening, talking and doing and the same coherent messages are drawn from each.

Kolb (1984) described how people learn:

- Experience: learning by involvement

- Reflective: learning by reviewing

- Generalisation/theorist: learning by reading and discussion

- Experiential or testing: learning through activities.

People can learn in many different ways, but by adulthood most people have demonstrated a preferred learning style. Nevertheless, learning involves several processes integrating activity with reflection, the discovery of new ideas and experimentation to see how our performance might be improved.

I will use the four points on the learning cycle as starting points for the learner – an entry point into the learning, not the place that they stay.

Fig. 1 Learning Cycle (after Kolb[2])

Everyday practice, for **the activist**, is the place to start. This is using the 20+ face to face consultations each working day and, as they are going on, thinking about the patients – why is this patient bringing these symptoms to me today?

Peter Tate, who managed the MRCGP panel so well for many years, described this as developing a curiosity about the patient. The way to find out is not lots of questions, but really active listening. The skills are listed in Figure 2, but the underlying skill is for the doctor to hear what the patient says and how they say it; then work out with the patient why they are saying it.

CHAPTER 3

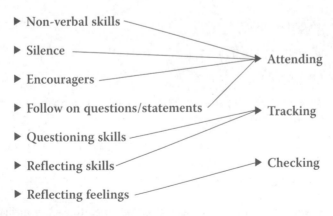

Fig. 2 Active listening

The **activist** can then use other aspects of the consultation to try new things and new ideas, but I am getting into the areas for the **experiential learner**.

The **reflective learner** might also start with the day-to-day consultation, but might wish to take the reflection further and use video feedback at an early stage. There are a number of published methods of doing this (Pendleton *et al* 2003[3]; Neighbour 1987[4]), but an easy place to start is using the COT criteria and getting help from the educational supervisor.

There is a lot of scope for the **generalist/theoretical learner** to start because the theoretical base of effective consulting is now vast and detailed. Probably, as suggested, the best starting place is the second chapter of the RCGP curriculum to get a simple overview; there is further reading indicated there. There are often articles in the current journals about different aspects of the consultation as it is of importance to all doctors regardless of their specialty. As well as reading discussion of cases with other clinicians, observing consultations can give an overview to the **generalist learner**.

The **experiential learner** will like to start with trying out new ideas in the consultation. These ideas might come from the trainer or from reading or discussion. There is a time and place to try out new skills: first thing Monday morning is probably not ideal. Introducing new skills needs planning:

- Start at a quiet time

- Be clear what you are trying to do

- Make small changes

- Don't be put off by the patient's initial reaction (it is probably new for them too and might need some explanation)

- Continue to practise a skill until it stops feeling awkward for you; get the words right until you feel comfortable with them

- Enjoy experimenting.

The reader will see from these starting points that there are artificial boundaries between the 'learning types'. It requires moving around the learning cycle many times and not staying in one area. Using all the opportunities within the training is essential to develop the skills to pass the CSA. Use the day release to get new approaches to the consultation and to get feedback from your peers; use the tutorials to cover areas that affect the consultation, eg when discussing diabetes ask your trainer how they manage the new patient with diabetes when informing them of the diagnosis. I have already mentioned COTs and along with the case-based discussion (CbD) they provide a rich source of feedback that can develop your consultations. Patient feedback and the results of your multi-source feedback (MSF) might give you pointers to develop your consultation skills. Your reading and discussions will give you skills and strategies that you might like to try in your consultations; make these into clear action plans and introduce them into your consultations.

Developing your consultation is like any skill that you might learn, eg learning the guitar or improving your wind-surfing. First, it is getting clarity about what it is you are trying to learn; second, trying it out and getting feedback on your performance, and third practising, practising and practising. The practice stage is often lost, and the improvement is not maintained. It is important when you practise to get the changes that you wish to make unconscious, so you don't need to keep trying to remember questions; they just come naturally.

SPECIFIC PREPARATION FOR THE CSA CONSULTATION SKILLS

As the time draws near for your CSA what is there to be done in the way of 'revision' or 'swotting'? It is really important to remember that, unlike written examinations, this is a test of clinical skills where the candidate needs to turn to the consulting room as a solid base of preparation. Use each and every consultation as a potential examination station: imagine that you are being observed and shed any incorrect or sloppy habits; follow up on clues presented, and hone your skills of reflection and analysis.

It is important at an early stage to encourage and welcome the more challenging consultations in your consulting room. Many doctors, particularly registrars, ignore clues that get them into difficult areas:

CHAPTER 3

Patient A   '... and I seem to be getting much more irritable recently.'

Doctor   ' Uh uh. How is your sleeping?'

Patient B   '... and it is very distressing.'

Doctor   'I wouldn't worry. It will be fine.'

Patient C   '... and since then I have felt so tired.'

Doctor   'I will do some blood tests to make sure that you are ok.'

All three of these patients have given the doctor clues that he has chosen to ignore. The doctor will say that they will ask the questions next time, but the next consultation is another occasion and the discussion will be about sleep patterns or blood test results. The moment will be lost when the possible responses could have been:

To patient A 'Tell me about the irritable feelings.'

To patient B 'Why is it distressing?'

To patient C 'Talk to me about this tiredness' or
                    'How did the tiredness start?'

Ignored cues in the day-to-day consultation are often lost forever and in the CSA they will lose the candidate marks.

IN THE EXAMINATION

It is important to treat every patient as though they are in your consulting room; be respectful and friendly. Stand up when you first meet the patient, welcome them and ensure that you address them by their name. Some patients may be blind, deaf or have other disabilities; they should be dealt with appropriately, guiding them or helping them to their seat if required. Do not 'show off' to the observer – that is a disaster. Interact with each patient appropriately even though the examination brief might be a clinical skill, eg examine the patient's knee and use those skills that you have been developing over your training:

- Really listen to the patient

- Make the history focused

- Make your explanations clear and jargon free, also succinct to save time – time is wasted by the doctor talking too much

- Check out understanding and ask for any questions

- Be aware of the patient's body language and react appropriately to it.

As well as being closely involved in the process of the consultation and using the above strategies and skills, it is important to have awareness of that process as it progresses:

- Be aware of the time

- Try to get a flow throughout each consultation

- Be logical and systematic.

Summarising the information that you have collected and checking it out with the patients are helpful ways of gathering your thoughts.

REFERENCES

1 Spence J (1960). The need for understanding the individual as part of the training and function of doctors and nurses. In: *The Purpose and Practice of Medicine*. Oxford: Oxford University Press, 271–280.

2 Kolb D (1984). *Experiential Learning: Experience as a source of learning and development.* Englewood Cliffs: Prentice Hall.

3 Pendleton D, Schofield T, Tate P, Havelock P (2003). *The New Consultation.* Oxford: Oxford University Press.

4 Neighbour R (1987). *The Inner Consultation: how to develop effective and intuitive consulting skills.* Lancaster: Kluwer Academic Press.

CHAPTER 3

Chapter 4
Exam Circuit 1

Case Number	1	2	3	4	5	6	7	8	9	10	11	12	13
The general practice consultation	✓	✓	✓	✓	✓	✓	✓	✓	✓	✓	✓	✓	✓
Clinical governance													
Patient safety	✓	✓	✓	✓	✓	✓	✓	✓	✓	✓	✓	✓	✓
Clinical ethics and values-based practice		✓		✓		✓		✓				✓	
Promoting equality and valuing diversity					✓		✓						✓
Evidence-based practice	✓	✓	✓			✓		✓		✓			✓
Research and academic activity													
Teaching, mentoring and clinical supervision													
Management in primary care													
Information management and technology		✓			✓			✓		✓			
Healthy people: promoting health and preventing disease		✓					✓			✓	✓		✓
Genetics in primary care	✓												
Care of acutely ill people						✓		✓		✓			
Care of children and young people									✓				
Care of older adults								✓				✓	✓
Women's health	✓					✓		✓					
Men's health				✓								✓	
Sexual health				✓									
Care of people with cancer and palliative care	✓												
Care of people with mental health problems			✓					✓	✓				
Care of people with learning disabilities													
Cardiovascular problems		✓						✓		✓	✓		
Digestive problems				✓									✓
Drug and alcohol problems													
ENT and facial problems			✓					✓					
Eye problems													
Metabolic problems				✓									
Neurological problems								✓				✓	
Respiratory problems													
Rheumatology and conditions of the musculoskeletal system (including trauma)				✓								✓	
Skin problems			✓	✓		✓							

Fig. 3 Circuit 1 cases plotted against RCGP curriculum

CASE 1

IN THIS STATION ...

You are a new doctor in the practice.

Tip

✓ Start a stopwatch now and give yourself 2 minutes to read through the case notes and brainstorm any points you may want to bring up during the consultation.

MATERIALS AND INSTRUCTIONS TO CANDIDATE (CASE NOTES)

Name	Sarah Morrison
Age	67 years
Address	11a The Mews, Great Kingshill, London NW5 2NF
Social and family history	Retired teacher
	Lives with husband, also a retired teacher
Past medical history	Hypertension
	Hysterectomy
Current medication	Amlodipine 5 mg od
Recent tests	TSH (thyroid-stimulating hormone): normal range
	Smear (age 64): no dyskaryosis

BRAINSTORM

Tip: make the most of the time you have before each consultation to brainstorm. Compose yourself; make notes about your consultation structure and the important points that you need to cover. Remember your consultation structure.

_____

_____

_____

_____

_____

_____

_____

_____

_____

_____

_____

_____

_____

_____

_____

_____

_____

_____

CHAPTER 4

EXAMINATION FINDINGS
Information offered on iPad if appropriate

No pallor

Slim build

Abdomen:

Appears distended

Generally tender

No discrete masses

No organomegaly

Ascites detected

Bowel sounds normal

Pelvic and rectal examination declined by patient

Urine dip: 3+ blood only

Respiratory:

Normal respiratory rate

Normal expansion, percussion note, fremitus and air entry

Peripheral oxygen saturations 97%

INSTRUCTIONS TO ROLE PLAYER (PATIENT OR CARER)

NOT TO BE SEEN BY THE CANDIDATE

You are Sarah Morrison, a 67-year-old retired teacher. You have been experiencing lower abdominal pain and bloating over the last few months. These symptoms have been getting worse recently and are now complicated by needing to pass urine more frequently.

You think you may have a urinary tract infection.

You're deeply worried about a sinister cause of the bloating and pain, but admit to this only if directly asked.

You decline any intimate examinations.

The doctor should explore the possibility of you having ovarian cancer.

Opening statement

[looking worried] 'Hello doctor, we've not met before. I think I may have a urinary tract infection.'

Freely divulged in response to open questions:

You have been passing urine more frequently for the last few months.

It doesn't burn or hurt when you pass urine although you have been experiencing lower abdominal pain for the last few months.

You're horrified at your dress size and feel embarrassed when you're with your husband.

You've brought a urine sample for the doctor to dip.

Information divulged if asked specifically:

For the past few months you've been passing urine about twice as often as you normally do. It doesn't hurt when you pass urine and there is no blood.

You have been a bit more constipated lately.

There is no blood or mucus in your stool.

You have not noticed any vaginal discharge or bleeding.

You had your hysterectomy when you were 40 because of heavy periods caused by fibroids. The gynaecologists didn't remove your ovaries.

Your pain is dull and in your lower abdomen.

The pain doesn't spread anywhere and is constant.

There are no exacerbating or relieving factors.

You feel bloated all the time and your skirts are getting tight; you've gone up three dress sizes. Your swollen abdomen feels like it's affecting your breathing, as though something is pressing on your diaphragm.

The pain doesn't disturb your sleep unless you turn in bed; it reminds you of being pregnant.

You feel unusually tired and have gained weight.

You're concerned that you have cancer of some form.

NOTES

OVERALL AIM OF THE CASE

The aim of this case is to explore beyond the surface; keep an open mind at the start of the consultation rather than accepting the patient's initial statement as the diagnosis.

DATA GATHERING, TECHNICAL AND ASSESSMENT SKILLS

- It's important to keep an open mind in the early stages of this consultation. It would be easy to be drawn into 'colluding' with the patient's opening statement and treating her for a urinary tract infection (UTI).

- She has had a hysterectomy; exploring whether this was ovary conserving is pivotal to this case. Making an assumption that it was a total hysterectomy and bilateral oophorectomy may cost this woman her life.

- Furthermore, she does have constipation, which may draw you into bowel pathology. This can be a symptom of ovarian cancer; a change towards looser stool tends to be suggestive of bowel cancer.

- Exploring and reflecting back why she thinks that she has a UTI will reveal her symptom complex and offer vital clues that this is not a case of a simple UTI, but is a probable ovarian tumour, eg she has a protracted history of urinary frequency and persistent abdominal bloating, and she does not experience dysuria.

- General observations on examination are helpful.

- An abdominal, pelvic and rectal examination is important. For the purposes of the CSA, personal examinations will not be permitted.

- Given the symptom of breathlessness, a chest examination, and arguably a cardiac examination, should also be performed. Given the time pressures within general practice, a cardiac examination is not essential.

CHAPTER 4

- A chest examination may reveal a pleural effusion, which may occur in the context of an ovarian tumour (eg Meigs syndrome: benign ovarian tumour, ascites, pleural effusion).

- The breathlessness may be caused by the pressure of the ascitic fluid splinting the diaphragm.

- It's possible that the examination findings are merely presented to you on the iPad rather than you having to perform a full examination.

CLINICAL MANAGEMENT SKILLS

- This patient has an ovarian tumour till proven otherwise.

- Urgent investigations including abdominal and pelvic ultrasound, and measurement of CA-125, are required.

- An MSU should still be sent for culture and sensitivity, and perhaps cytology.

- The ultrasound scan will confirm ascites and should offer a vital clue as to its cause. Remember that the differential of ascites is wide and includes cor pulmonale, tuberculosis (TB), pancreatitis, intra-abdominal tumours and metastatic disease.

- Remember that there are several causes of a raised CA-125 level.

- Robust safety netting and urgent follow-up are required

INTERPERSONAL SKILLS

- A clear logical approach with regular summarising is important to ensure that you understand the patient and that the patient understands you and feels listened to.

- The patient is looking worried; exploration of this cue may reveal the concern of a malignancy and she may feel enabled to vocalise more symptoms.

- Empathy is required.

- It's important not to falsely reassure but to assure that you will investigate quickly.

CHAPTER 4

- What are her expectations? Manage expectations, eg what and why you're organising investigations, what an ultrasound is and what may happen next, ie 2-week wait (2WW) referral, CT (computed tomography) scan.

- Offer hope, if the conversation arises, that this may not be cancer and that it may benign. If it is cancer, it may be treatable.

- Be honest that there are a lot of unknowns.

KEY POINTS

- Ovarian cancer is the fourth most common cause of cancer death in the UK

- Often diagnosed too late

- Risk factors:

  - Advancing age

  - Low parity

  - Early menarche

  - Late menopause

  - *BRCA*

- Features that should raise suspicion of ovarian cancer:

  - Persistent abdominal bloating

  - Early satiety

  - Abdominal/pelvic pain

  - Urinary frequency/urgency

  - Change in bowel habit

  - Features of IBS (irritable bowel syndrome) in a woman aged >50 years

- Causes of a raised CA-125:

  - Malignant: ovary, endometrial, cervical, breast, hepatocellular, pancreas, colon, lung, lymphoma

  - Non-malignant: endometriosis, fibroids, pregnancy, hepatitis, liver disease, ascites, pancreatitis, IBD (inflammatory bowel disease), peritonitis, urinary retention, osteoarthritis, rheumatoid arthritis, SLE (systemic lupus erythematosus), chronic kidney disease, cystic fibrosis, diabetes mellitus, diverticulitis, IBS, heart failure, pericarditis, pneumonia.

FURTHER READING

Cancer Research UK has a very good summary on ovarian cancer.

Clinical review – Ovarian cancer, *GPonline*, 2012. www.gponline.com/Clinical/article/1130709/Clinical-Review---Ovarian-cancer. This is a comprehensive overview on ovarian cancer.

MIMS Consultation Guide for extensive list of differential diagnoses, explanation of tests and disease summaries – an excellent revision aid.

CHAPTER 4

CASE 2

IN THIS STATION ...

You are a locum GP in the practice.

MATERIALS AND INSTRUCTIONS TO CANDIDATE (CASE NOTES)

Name	Tony Parsons
Age	78 years
Address	101 Newlands Flats, Bloomsbury Gardens, London W1
Social and family history	Lives with wife, Brenda
	Smoker
Past medical history	STEMI (ST-elevation myocardial infarction) in 2009
	Hypertension
	Hypercholesterolaemia
Current medication	Aspirin 75 mg od (alert: under-use)
	Ramipril 5 mg od
	Bisoprolol 5 mg od
	Amlodipine 5 mg od
	Atorvastatin 40 mg od
Last cholesterol (3 months ago)	4.0 mmol/l

BRAINSTORM

EXAMINATION FINDINGS
Information offered on iPad if appropriate

Sinus rhythm 60 beats/min

BP 158/68 mmHg

Bilateral carotid bruits

Neurological examination normal

INSTRUCTIONS TO ROLE PLAYER (PATIENT OR CARER)

NOT TO BE SEEN BY THE CANDIDATE

You are Tony Parsons, a 78-year-old retired policeman. You've had a stressful career working in the murder squad.

You think you had a mini-stroke yesterday evening. You couldn't speak for about 20 minutes.

You've come to the doctor without your wife, worried and asking for help.

Opening statement:

'Hello doctor, I think I had a mini-stroke last night; my wife saw the whole thing but she couldn't make it today.'

Freely divulged in response to open questions:

You were watching TV last night and chatting to your wife when your speech suddenly changed.

Your words came out all jumbled.

You thought that you were having a stroke.

Everything went back to normal after 20 minutes.

Information divulged if asked specifically:

You've never experienced this before.

You tried to talk and it came out like a foreign language.

You didn't experience any weakness in your limbs.

You didn't lose consciousness.

You're aware that this was a mini-stroke and that a stroke is like a 'brain attack' and should be taken seriously.

You had no idea that this may herald a major stroke.

You take drugs to lower your cholesterol and blood pressure, hence you thought that you would be immune from getting further cardiovascular disease; because of this you continue to smoke. Your wife cooks healthy foods, but you often eat chips and chocolate behind her back.

You take your medicines as prescribed, except for aspirin; you just decided, because the dose seemed so small, that it wasn't that important.

You checked your blood sugar at the chemist last week and were told that it was normal.

You enjoy smoking but are willing to change your lifestyle if advised.

You're happy to take whatever advice the doctor gives you.

You're worried what might happen in hospital.

NOTES

OVERALL AIM OF THE CASE

This case is about managing the patient's health beliefs, and recognising and managing a TIA (transient ischaemic attack) as a risk factor for major stroke.

DATA GATHERING, TECHNICAL AND ASSESSMENT SKILLS

- A clear understanding of what the patient experienced is essential.

- It is important to establish the diagnosis and its severity, and if possible consider potential sources of emboli, eg AF (atrial fibrillation)/carotid artery stenosis/atrial septal defect.

- Conformation that there are no residual neurological anomalies will rule out a stroke (it is quite possible that the examination findings will be given to you in the CSA rather than expecting you to have to perform one).

- In this case, there are no abnormal neurological signs; the patient is in sinus rhythm and has carotid bruits. Note that patients in sinus rhythm may have paroxysmal AF which carries the same stroke risk as persistent/permanent AF.

- NICE (National Institute for Health and Care Excellence) endorses the ABCD2 risk score in patients with a TIA, and questions should cover this.

- It is important to establish whether he has had any other TIA episodes previously. Two low-risk TIAs in the last week should be considered high risk overall.

- The ABCD2 score in this case: 4

CHAPTER 4

CLINICAL MANAGEMENT SKILLS

- Aspirin 300 mg od should be commenced.

- Refer for further assessment at a local TIA clinic to be seen within 24 hours because the ABCD2 score is 4.

- Advice on drug adherence.

- Smoking cessation advice and referral to a smoking cessation counsellor if patient agrees.

- Offer lifestyle counselling and advice on driving.

- Clear safety net.

- Follow-up after the hospital appointment will include a blood pressure check.

INTERPERSONAL SKILLS

- Recognise that this may be a frightening experience and address any concerns.

- Explain what is going on in language that the patient understands. Summarise and check understanding at points throughout the consultation.

- Explore if the patient has expectations, and manage them accordingly.

- Don't be judgemental re smoking and drug adherence with aspirin, but emphasise the importance of prevention and healthy living.

KEY POINTS

ABCD scoring system		
Age	>60 years	1 point
	<60 years	0 points
Blood pressure	>140/90 mmHg	1 point
	<140/90 mmHg	0 points
Clinical features	Speech impairment without weakness	1 point
	Unilateral weakness	2 points
Duration	10–59 min	1 point
	>60 min	2 points
Diabetes mellitus	Yes	1 point

Reproduced with kind permission of GPonline.

- Score of ≥4, or two or more TIAs in the last week, require specialist assessment within 24 hours.

- Scores of ≤3 should be assessed within 7 days

FURTHER READING

www.nice.org.uk covers the latest advice on stroke and TIAs.

Identifying and managing TIAs. *GPonline*, 2010. www.gponline.com/Clinical/article/1033895/Identifying-managing-TIA. This article gives a comprehensive overview of TIAs – recognition and management.

CHAPTER 4

CASE 3

IN THIS STATION ...

You are a GP in a busy clinic.

MATERIALS AND INSTRUCTIONS TO CANDIDATE (CASE NOTES)

Name	Jason King
Age	45 years
Address	18 Drayton Close, Chalk Farm, London NW5 3AD
Social and family history	Lorry driver
	Lives with wife and three children
Past medical history	Psoriasis
Current medication	Calcipotriol
	Betacap

Examination of patient's thumb:

BRAINSTORM

INSTRUCTIONS TO ROLE PLAYER (PATIENT OR CARER)

You are Jason King, a lorry driver, and have come to see the doctor about your nails.

Your previous GP felt that it was a fungal infection, but, as you were moving to this current practice, she didn't want to initiate treatment.

All your nails are discoloured and you're convinced that it's due to a fungal infection because your stepfather has fungally infected toenails.

You want the antifungal tablets that your stepfather is taking.

You have no idea that your nail disease is due to psoriasis rather than a fungal infection.

Opening statement:

'Hi doc, I think I need some treatment for my fungal nail infection.'

Freely divulged in response to open questions:

All finger and toenails are affected.

They have been like this for many years.

They are not painful and crumble easily.

Information divulged if asked specifically:

Your skin and scalp psoriasis is well controlled.

You're convinced that the problem is caused by a fungal infection and would like drugs for this.

You've tried over-the-counter, 'paint-on' medication with no improvement.

You're surprised to hear that the nail disease could be due to psoriasis.

You don't really understand what psoriasis is.

You're not overly keen to wait for nail clippings to be sent to the lab and would prefer to try antifungal medication.

You didn't realise that the medication can have serious side effects and agree to have samples sent to the lab; if the samples are negative for fungal elements you're willing to see a dermatologist.

You're embarrassed about your nails and this has affected your confidence; you're not depressed.

CHAPTER 4

NOTES

OVERALL AIM OF THE CASE

To manage patient's health beliefs, recognise the psychological consequences of disease and manage it accordingly.

DATA GATHERING, TECHNICAL AND ASSESSMENT SKILLS

> ✓ **When approaching new problems, it's useful to consider the differential diagnosis of the symptom and ask questions accordingly. Explaining the differential to the patient signals your logical approach and keeps them involved and engaged.**

- There are several causes of onycholysis including congenital, infection (fungal, *Pseudomonas* sp.), psoriasis, trauma, sarcoid and amyloid. Care needs to be taken not to miss a melanoma.

- Given that he has a history of psoriasis, it's highly likely to be psoriatic nail disease.

- It's important to explore whether any chronic or disfiguring condition is affecting a patient's mental health.

- Checking whether his skin psoriasis is under control is good practice.

CLINICAL MANAGEMENT SKILLS

- It would be usual to send adequate nail samples for mycology.

- Psoriatic nails, particularly when widespread or causing distress, should be referred to a dermatologist.

- Manage the psychosocial impact of the disease.

INTERPERSONAL SKILLS

- Exploring the patient's health beliefs and offering education are important and empowering for the patient. Signposting to websites is often useful, eg www.psoriasis-association.org.uk and www.bad.org.uk.

- Education on what psoriasis is will again empower the patient and help him manage his condition more effectively.

- Summarising and checking understanding will make the patient feel valued.

- Recognising that his condition may affect his confidence will forge a good therapeutic relationship.

KEY POINTS

- Psoriasis: 1–3% prevalence (European population)

- Aetiology and risk factors: family history, infections (bacterial, HIV, scabies) stress, obesity, smoking, alcohol, drugs (lithium, β blockers)

- Subtypes:

  - *Chronic plaque:* 90% cases, large well-demarcated plaques, pink with silvery scale, often on extensor surfaces

  - *Guttate:* children/teenagers, post-β-haemolytic streptococcal/viral infection, small plaques over trunk

  - *Generalised pustular:* fever, malaise, unwell, pustules

  - *Palmoplantar pustular:* F > M; pustules noted on palms and soles

- Complications: arthropathy, nail involvement (50%, pitting, onycholysis, nails may be affected without skin disease), scalp disease, alopecia, secondary bacterial infection, depression, low self-esteem, suicide, erythroderma

- Nail disease is associated with, and is more severe with, psoriatic arthritis

CHAPTER 4

55

- Management:

  - *Chronic plaque psoriasis*: vitamin D analogues (first line but too irritant for face), emollients, combination vitamin D analogues/ betamethasone (not for maintenance), topical steroids, topical tar agents (cause staining), coal-tar bath additives, topical retinoids for very scaly lesions, dithranol, salicylic acid with steroids or white, soft paraffin. Review after 4–6 weeks.

  - *Scalp psoriasis:* vitamin D/betamethasone combination, steroid shampoo/lotion/gel, coconut compounds for scaly disease, tar shampoo (adjunct or for mild scalp disease)

  - *Erythrodermic*: secondary care, fluids, topical agents, immunosuppressants, infliximab, UVB, PUVA (psoralen + UVA), analgesia

  - *Generalised pustular*: urgent referral required.

  - *Palmoplantar pustular*: often requires systemic treatment; psychodermatology

  - *Second-line agents:* tacrolimus/pimecrolimus, UVB, PUVA, methotrexate, azathioprine, ciclosporin, hydroxyurea

  - *Third-line agents:* eg infliximab, etanercept, adalimumab, ustekinumab.

  - *Guttate:* often resolves spontaneously.

  - Ensure compliance.

FURTHER READING

The latest NICE guidelines on psoriasis were published in October 2012.

CHAPTER 4

CASE 4

IN THIS STATION ...

You are a new GP in the practice.

MATERIALS AND INSTRUCTIONS TO CANDIDATE (CASE NOTES)

Name	Harriet Green
Age	38 years
Address	23 Holtspur Close, Euston Wharf, London W1
Social and family history	Personal assistant to Chief Executive Officer, Biopharm Ltd
	Married a year ago
Past medical history	Tennis elbow
	Shingles
	Hypothyroidism
Current medication	Levothyroxine 100 mcg od
On examination of patient's face	Erythematous symmetrical butterfly rash

CHAPTER 4

BRAINSTORM

INSTRUCTIONS TO ROLE PLAYER (PATIENT OR CARER)

You're Harriet Green, a 38-year-old personal assistant to a large biotech company.

You've had a rash on your face for around a year.

Your last GP said that it was shingles and you'd like to try aciclovir again; it hadn't worked in the past.

You've also been treated for rosacea with no improvement.

The rash is deeply upsetting and damaging your self-esteem

Opening statement:

'Hello doctor, about my rash, I'd like to try aciclovir.'

Freely divulged in response to open questions:

You've had the rash for a year.

It came on 'out of the blue'.

Your last GP was convinced it was shingles and gave aciclovir, which didn't work.

Another GP then tried several treatments for rosacea, with no improvement.

You'd like to give the aciclovir another go.

Information divulged if asked specifically:

You are a little sceptical about a diagnosis of shingles; you've not seen any blisters and you remember being told shingles isn't symmetrical – yours is. However, you would give any treatment a chance, including another course of aciclovir.

You've tried lymecycline, erythromycin and topical metronidazole for rosacea with no benefit.

The joints in your hands have been painful over the last few months.

You've never heard of lupus.

The rash is damaging your confidence. You feel your new husband has avoided sex recently because of the rash and you feel lonely. Life is worth living and you're not depressed.

CHAPTER 4

NOTES

OVERALL AIM OF THE CASE

To challenge diagnoses given by previous doctors, discuss a potential new serious diagnosis and investigate accordingly.

DATA GATHERING, TECHNICAL AND ASSESSMENT SKILLS

- In this case, it is important to understand the nature of the rash, eg distribution, onset, associated symptoms.

- Rashes of this nature have several causes but the most likely two to exclude are rosacea and lupus.

- Once you have formulated your differential diagnoses, questions should be asked accordingly.

- The symmetrical distribution, absence of blisters and lack of pain exclude shingles.

- Given that she has tried several treatments for rosacea, all of which have failed, that is also less likely.

- If, by history taking, your working diagnosis is lupus, asking questions to refute or corroborate your theory is helpful.

- In her case, she has joint pains, which fit with lupus.

CLINICAL MANAGEMENT SKILLS

- It wouldn't be unreasonable at this stage to arrange serological blood tests that would point towards lupus.

- You also wouldn't be criticised if you referred the patient to a dermatologist, except to say that, if your bloods turn out to be positive for lupus, you may have wasted a dermatology appointment because the patient may have been referred directly to a rheumatologist; in the new age of commissioning, this could be considered a poor use of resources.

- Asking a dermatologist for advice, perhaps sending a picture (with consent), would be innovative and appropriate.
- Follow-up is important.

INTERPERSONAL SKILLS

- It's important to recognise the psychological consequences, pick up on cues and give hope.
- Be clear to the patient that the diagnosis may be, but is not definitely, lupus so that expectations are managed.
- Ensure that the patient understands your language and thought process by intermittently summarising and checking understanding. This is important when discussing a potential new and complex diagnosis.
- Explore health beliefs and offering education will empower the patient.

KEY POINTS

- Systemic lupus erythematosus affects females more than males.
- Peak onset 15-40 years.
- Risk factors: autoimmune, genetic, drugs, Klinefelter syndrome.
- Clinical features: fever, malaise, fatigue, skin (photosensitive facial butterfly rash, vasculitis, scarring alopecia, Raynaud phenomenon, livedo reticularis, subcutaneous nodules, bullae, discoid lupus, telangiectasia), joint pains (non-erosive arthritis [Jaccoud arthropathy], deformity), muscle pains, oral ulceration.
- Complications: CNS (headaches, psychosis, seizures), pleural effusions, cardiac (pericarditis, pericardial effusions, myocarditis, Libman–Sacks endocarditis, accelerated congestive heart failure, myocardial infarction [MI]), renal (glomerulonephritis, nephritic

CHAPTER 4

syndrome, proteinuria, haematuria), haematological (anaemia of chronic disease, haemolysis, lymphadenopathy, splenomegaly), eyes (sicca syndrome, haemorrhages, papilloedema), miscarriage, VTE (venous thromboembolism).

- Usual cause of death: renal failure, cardiovascular disease, infections.

- Management: education, refer urgently if cardiorenal involvement, UV light, sunblock, hydroxychloroquine (with annual optician review), systemic steroids for flare, methotrexate, azathioprine, cyclophosphamide, rituximab, mycophenolate mofetil, cardiorenal risk assessment (maintain blood pressure [BP] <130/80 mmHg), low-dose aspirin for pregnant women.

CASE 5

IN THIS STATION ...

You are a salaried GP at the practice.

MATERIALS AND INSTRUCTIONS TO CANDIDATE (CASE NOTES)

Name	Jerry Smith
Age	47 years
Address	123 Huntley Street, London W1
Social and family history	Architect
	Lives with partner, Steven
Past medical history	Nil
Current medication	Nil

CHAPTER 4

BRAINSTORM

EXAMINATION FINDINGS

Information offered on iPad if appropriate

Slim

Afebrile

Sweaty palms

Fine tremor

Pulse 120 regular

BM 5.7 mmol/l

Chest clear, no murmurs, no abnormalities detected on abdomen

INSTRUCTIONS TO ROLE PLAYER (PATIENT OR CARER)

You are Jerry Smith, a shy architect working in London.

For the past 8 weeks you've been losing weight and been sweatier than usual.

You're gay and are worried about HIV.

Opening statement:

'Hello doctor, we've not met before. I've been losing weight. I probably ought to tell you I'm gay.'

Freely divulged in response to open questions:

You've been losing weight for 2 months, about half a stone (3 kg).

You've no idea why it's been happening.

Information divulged if asked specifically:

You're normally fit and well.

You're eating more than usual and eat a healthy and balanced diet. You're not vegetarian.

Your bowels are looser than normal but there is no blood.

You're not thirsty nor do you pass urine more than usual.

You're sweatier than normal, throughout the day and night.

You are worried that you may have HIV, given that you slept with a man without protection at a party a few months back. You've not been tested for HIV because you've been with your partner for 6 years. You feel remorse re this and have never been unfaithful either before or since.

You don't have any other symptoms.

You're not depressed. You only drink at Christmas and you don't take drugs.

NOTES

OVERALL AIM OF THE CASE

To be able to establish a diagnosis from a wide possible list of differentials and put the case in the context of the patient's life in a sensitive manner.

DATA GATHERING, TECHNICAL AND ASSESSMENT SKILLS

- As with most new symptoms, building a quick list of differentials in your mind and asking questions in logical order will help avoid missing an important diagnosis.

- Weight loss can be suggestive of poor diet, poor absorption or hypermetabolic states.

- Mr Smith eats well. Coeliac disease or an inflamed bowel may cause malabsorption whereas excess calorie expenditure may suggest malignancy, infection or thyroid disease

- The social history is important here and his HIV (human immunodeficiency virus) risk needs to be explored.

- A review of symptoms to exclude any red flags for malignancy and infection such as TB and endocarditis is important and demonstrates safe practice to the examiner.

- A thyroid and general systems examination should be offered.

CLINICAL MANAGEMENT SKILLS

- Urgent thyroid function tests (TFTs), HIV test and coeliac bloods are very reasonable tests to perform. An FBC is also justified.

- Given the sweats and weight loss, a chest radiograph would not be unreasonable.

- You may wish to express that you would like to check a BM (blood glucose) in clinic.

CHAPTER 4

- Clear safety netting and robust follow-up are essential.

INTERPERSONAL SKILLS

- Explaining your differentials early in the consultation and that you would like to ask questions accordingly will keep the patient on board and give him confidence.

- Sensitivity is required, particularly given that HIV is an emotive subject.

- He will also be concerned, if he does have HIV, that he may have passed it to his partner.

- It is important not to appear judgemental or 'thrown' by the fact that this patient may have HIV.

- Explaining what tests you are doing and why helps to keep the patient on board and reassures him.

KEY POINTS

The differential diagnosis for weight loss is wide and includes: malnutrition, malabsorption, hyperthyroidism, depression, mania, malignancy, alcoholism, poorly controlled/undiagnosed diabetes mellitus, chronic infection (TB, endocarditis, HIV, parasitic infections), Addison disease, cystic fibrosis, Parkinson's disease, dementia, connective tissue diseases, iatrogenic (eg ACE [angiotensin-converting enzyme] inhibitors, amiodarone, amphetamines, metformin, levodopa, calcitriol, bicalutamide, clonazepam, clonidine, thyroxine, digoxin, donepezil, SSRIs [selective serotonin reuptake inhibitors], leflunomide, NSAIDs [non-steroidal anti-inflammatory drugs], topiramate, zidovudine).

FURTHER READING

Thakkar R. *The MIMS Consultation Guide*. 2011.

CHAPTER 4

CASE 6

IN THIS STATION ...

You are a locum GP, and have been asked to call a patient on the telephone regarding her urine dipstick results.

MATERIALS AND INSTRUCTIONS TO CANDIDATE (CASE NOTES)

Name	Jessica Thompson
Age	23 years
Address	3 Chalford Flats, Wooburn Street, Hallstead, London NW9 3ST
Social and family history	Waitress
	Lives with parents
Past medical history	Psoriasis
	Erythema multiforme
Current medication	Methotrexate 10 mg/week
	Folic acid 5 mg/week
	Ethinylestradiol 30 mcg/levonorgestrel 150 mcg as per pill cycle
Urine results	Positive for leukocytes, nitrites, protein and blood

BRAINSTORM

INSTRUCTIONS TO ROLE PLAYER (PATIENT OR CARER)

You are Jessica Thompson, a 23-year-old waitress.

For the last 24 hours you have been experiencing burning when you pass urine and think that you may have a urine infection. In the last hour, you've started to feel unwell, have developed pain over your left kidney and feel feverish.

You dropped in a urine sample to the surgery this morning for the doctor to dip.

Opening statement:

'Hello doctor, have you checked my urine?'

Freely divulged in response to open questions:

You have experienced burning, frequency and urgency of urine over the last 24 hours.

You're sure that you have a urine infection.

You would like some antibiotics, especially as you're going on holiday the day after tomorrow and want to be well. You initially don't want to come to the surgery but will if the doctor persuades you.

Information divulged if asked specifically:

For the last hour you've felt more unwell, and developed a fever, sweatiness and pain in the left-hand side of your back, where your kidney is.

You feel dizzy and have just experienced a severe shaking episode that lasted under a minute.

You wonder whether you have a kidney infection and you would like to come into the surgery.

Your last period finished a week ago and you haven't had sex since then.

You're allergic to nitrofurantoin – you had a urine infection years ago and had a nasty rash with this.

CHAPTER 4

You have psoriasis and take methotrexate for that. You're aware that you're more prone to infection. You are also aware that you should not have a drug called trimethoprim because you take methotrexate, but you're unsure why.

You can take penicillin.

You live at home with your parents.

Your dad can bring you to the surgery at any time; you live only 5 minutes away.

CHAPTER 4

NOTES

OVERALL AIM OF THE CASE

To explore what seemed to be a simple UTI but was in fact pyelonephritis. To manage a potentially serious condition safely over the telephone.

DATA GATHERING, TECHNICAL AND ASSESSMENT SKILLS

- Telephone consultations require detailed questioning to ensure that the patient is not at risk.

- In this case, unless the patient is asked specifically, pyelonephritis and potential sepsis may be missed.

- It is important to ask for typical features of cystitis and whether there are any features of an upper UTI and septicaemia.

- Her drug history is crucial to avoid errors and interactions.

CLINICAL MANAGEMENT SKILLS

- This patient has pyelonephritis with possible sepsis.

- She needs a face-to-face assessment quickly and may need admission.

- Offering her antibiotics over the phone would be acceptable only if she had simple cystitis.

- Trimethoprim is not appropriate for pyelonephritis and should not be used with methotrexate because both drugs are folate antagonists.

- Nitrofurantoin is contraindicated with her due to a history of erythema multiforme and is for use only in cystitis.

- The sample should be sent to the lab for culture and sensitivity.

CHAPTER 4

INTERPERSONAL SKILLS

- It is important not to panic her but, at the same time, ensure that she attends for a face-to-face assessment

- Explaining the clinical importance of a face-to-face assessment helps to persuade her to come in for an assessment

KEY POINTS

Antibiotic therapy in UTIs (adults).

Acute pyelonephritis	Ciprofloxacin 500mg bd for 7 days		Follow local antibiotic policies. Review treatment when culture results available
	Co-amoxiclav 500/125mg tds for 14 days		
	In pregnancy: Cefalexin 500mg bd for 10–14 days		
Uncomplicated lower UTI	Trimethoprim 200mg bd for 3 or 7 days in women and 7 days in men, pregnancy or indwelling catheter		Review treatment when urine culture results available
	Nitrofurantoin 50mg qds (or 100mg modified release bd) for 3 days in women and 7 days in men, pregnancy or indwelling catheter		

Reproduced with kind permission of MIMS.

CHAPTER 4

CASE 7

IN THIS STATION ...

You are a new doctor at the practice where the CCG (clinical commissioning group) considers seborrhoeic warts as cosmetic and their removal is not commissioned.

MATERIALS AND INSTRUCTIONS TO CANDIDATE (CASE NOTES)

Name	David Barclay
Age	58 years
Address	Cherry Farm, Hambledon, Hampstead, London NW9
Social and family history	Company director
	Lives with wife and three children
Past medical history	Hypertension
	Benign prostatic hyperplasia
	Splenectomy
Current medication	Amlodipine 5 mg od
	Tamsulosin M/R 400 mcg od
Patient's skin lesion	Typical seborrhoeic wart

Examination of patient's skin lesion:

BRAINSTORM

_____

_____

_____

_____

_____

_____

_____

_____

_____

_____

_____

_____

_____

_____

_____

_____

_____

_____

_____

_____

CHAPTER 4

INSTRUCTIONS TO ROLE PLAYER (PATIENT OR CARER)

You are David Barclay, a company director

You have a skin lesion on your chest and you would like an NHS referral to get it removed. You threaten to complain to the GMC (General Medical Council) unless you get a referral, but eventually calm down once you realise the difficulty that the NHS is in.

Opening statement:

'Hello doctor, my name is Mr Barclay; I'd like a referral for my skin please.'

Freely divulged in response to open questions:

You've had the skin lesion for a year.

Your wife finds it repulsive and you want a referral to get it removed.

Another GP has told you that the lesion is a seborrhoeic wart and the NHS won't pay for its removal.

You pay more than enough tax and your children attend private school; you think that deserves an NHS referral.

Information divulged if asked specifically:

You've had the lesion for years; it's barely changed over time.

It doesn't itch or bleed.

You showed it to a friend who is a plastic surgeon; he suggested that you get a referral from the GP. Your previous GP said that the local commissioning group won't pay for it because it's considered cosmetic.

You don't have any moles.

There is no family history of melanoma.

You've never used a sun bed.

You admit that you don't know much about the state of the NHS and why you can't get the referral.

No matter what the GP says, you don't change your view about the referral; however, afterwards you concede that it's a stalemate and will go privately to have the lesion taken off.

You know that you should take daily penicillin after your splenectomy – it was removed after a rugby accident. You don't actually know why it's so important to take the penicillin.

You're willing to take penicillin now that you realise its importance.

NOTES

OVERALL AIM OF THE CASE

To be able to manage and withstand challenge from a patient and to be inquisitive about a patient's past medical history.

DATA GATHERING, TECHNICAL AND ASSESSMENT SKILLS

- Although this is a 'spot diagnosis' it is nevertheless important to take a robust history so that you can defend and justify your actions.

- Questions about length of time that the lesion has been present, and checking whether the patient has experienced itching and bleeding, are relevant.

- Equally, exclusion of red flags to exclude melanomas according to the ABCDE rule (*a*symmetry, *b*order, *c*olour, *d*iameter, *e*volution) is relevant. Note that seborrhoeic warts can sometimes look like melanomas, in which case referral is justified.

- Being inquisitive about why he had a splenectomy shows interest and can improve his health, eg exploring why he isn't taking prophylactic penicillin.

CLINICAL MANAGEMENT SKILLS

- Removal of skin lesion is not commissioned by the local CCG and therefore will not be paid for by the NHS.

- A private referral may be offered.

- Prophylactic penicillin should be suggested based on the increased risk of infection from capsulated organisms such as those that cause meningococcal disease.

CHAPTER 4

INTERPERSONAL SKILLS

- This type of conversation may become all too common in the world of commissioning.

- Skills are required to educate the patient about the system and how it is resource based while maintaining a doctor–patient relationship.

- GPs now have a responsibility to spend public money wisely.

- Recognition of his situation and frustration can be helpful.

KEY POINTS

- The structure of general practice changed in April 2013, with all GPs becoming commissioners of services that they effectively purchase within an allocated budget.

- All GPs are members of CCGs.

- CCGs are statutory bodies and are 'headed up' by a board of clinical and non-clinical directors and their teams.

- The significant clinical presence in the leadership team of the CCG means that it has a huge insight into what happens on the 'front line' and can influence fellow clinicians far more easily than the old primary care trusts (PCTs).

- The CCG will commission services from providers such as hospitals or other establishments.

- Given that GPs are providers of medical care as well as commissioners, their contract is with the local area team (LAT), rather than the CCG, which is part of NHS England. This is because GPs are members of the CCG already and can't be providers of the services that they commission; this would be a conflict of interest.

- The agenda of the CCG is to commission and develop high-quality services, to reduce waste in the system, and to develop and innovate to ensure that the CCG stays in budget.

- Not removing seborrhoeic warts is an example of CCG policy (and probably old PCT policy), given that removal serves nothing but a cosmetic function and isn't a good use of a finite public purse.

CASE 8

IN THIS STATION ...

You are the duty GP at the local practice.

MATERIALS AND INSTRUCTIONS TO CANDIDATE (CASE NOTES)

Name	Betty Arnold
Age	78 years
Address	89 Meare Estate, Camden Town, London N5
Social and family history	Husband died last year
	Lives on own
Past medical history	Osteoarthritis
	Depression
Current medication	Paracetamol 500 mg 2 qds
	Sertraline 50 mg od
Consultation (2 days ago)	Depression (new)
	Depressed since death of husband. Low mood few months, poor sleep and appetite, has lost some weight. Not suicidal. Biophysical profile completed (see scanned doc). Moderately inactive. HAD (Hospital Anxiety and Depression scale) score 18/21 (depression); 14/21 (anxiety)
	o/e poor eye contact, no psychotic features

Plan: options discussed, for sertraline 50 mg od and review 2–3 weeks. Lifestyle counselling

CHAPTER 4

BRAINSTORM

EXAMINATION FINDINGS

Information offered on iPad if appropriate

Pulse: 80 beats/min sinus rhythm

Lying BP: 124/70 mmHg

Standing BP: 90/40 mmHg

Normal heart sounds

INSTRUCTIONS TO ROLE PLAYER (PATIENT OR CARER)

You are Betty Arnold, aged 78. Your husband died from a stroke last year.

This was devastating for you.

You saw a GP earlier this week who diagnosed depression. You were commenced on sertraline.

Since taking it you've felt very dizzy. You don't find it easy to explain what exactly you mean by 'dizzy'.

Opening statement:

'Hello doctor, have you read my notes? I've not felt well since starting those antidepressants.'

Freely divulged in response to open questions:

You started antidepressants 2 days ago.

Since taking them you've felt very dizzy.

You nearly fell over yesterday.

You don't want to take any more medication.

Information divulged if asked specifically:

The room doesn't spin; it's not like being on a boat.

You feel very light-headed on standing.

You haven't experienced any palpitations.

You haven't passed out but you feel like you might.

Your speech is fine and you haven't experienced any limb weakness.

You're cross because you feel that the GP should have warned you about the side effects.

You're willing to take half the current strength of sertraline (25 mg od).

Your daughter can stay with you and look after you if need be; she's in the waiting room.

CHAPTER 4

NOTES

OVERALL AIM OF THE CASE

To be able to use history taking to establish the most likely cause of a new symptom, risk stratify and negotiate with the patient.

DATA GATHERING, TECHNICAL AND ASSESSMENT SKILLS

- Dizziness can be complicated and it's important to be clear about what the patient is experiencing.
- Excluding vertigo excludes several underlying causes, whereas establishing that she is experiencing postural symptoms should create a particular list of differential diagnoses.
- In this case, once it is established that the patient is experiencing postural symptoms, questions need to be asked accordingly.
- In particular, the symptoms started only after sertraline 50 mg od.
- This is a high starting dose in elderly people.
- The examination should confirm postural hypotension, but also ensure that there is no cardiac arrhythmia or aortic stenosis.

CLINICAL MANAGEMENT SKILLS

- It would be reasonable to halve the dose of sertraline to 25 mg od, if the patient is agreeable.
- Ensuring that she is not home alone provides an extra tier of safety.
- Appropriate safety netting is essential.
- Follow-up should be arranged.

CHAPTER 4

INTERPERSONAL SKILLS

- Asking questions in a way that the patient understands is crucial; summarising and checking understanding at various points provide natural breaks in the consultation.

- It is easy to become frustrated if the patient finds it difficult to articulate what he or she is experiencing; don't let this show. Furthermore, putting pressure on the patient to 'perform' better will only make matters worse.

- Try not to get drawn into criticising colleagues; at the same time, telling the patient that you will discuss the case with the GP who prescribed the sertraline may offer some reassurance.

KEY POINTS

Although this case was on a presyncopal patient rather than syncope, the principles below are still important:

- Syncope is classified by the European Society of Cardiology into three subtypes: reflex, orthostatic hypotension and cardiac.

- Reflex syncope (most common) includes vasovagal (triggers include pain and fear; situational, such as coughing and post-micturition; and carotid sinus hypersensitivity).

- Orthostatic hypotension includes autonomic neuropathy (eg diabetes mellitus, Parkinson's disease), drugs and hypovolaemia.

- Cardiac syncope may be subdivided into arrhythmia, structural heart disease including aortic stenosis, cardiomyopathy and tumours, and others, such as aortic dissection, pulmonary embolus and pulmonary hypertension.

- Risk stratification is important given the inherent risks of injury and sudden cardiac death in syncopal patients with structural heart disease and conduction defects.

- Psychiatric disease may be considered in some cases and a diagnosis of pseudo-syncope may be made.

CHAPTER 4

- Treatment depends on the state of the patient, the underlying cause and if the patient is high risk.

FURTHER READING

See Thakkar, R. *The Basics – managing syncope*, 201. Available at: www. gponline.com/Clinical/article/1063707/Basics---Managing-syncope.

CHAPTER 4

CASE 9

IN THIS STATION ...

You are a new GP at the local practice.

MATERIALS AND INSTRUCTIONS TO CANDIDATE (CASE NOTES)

Name	Sarah Fountain
Age	34 years
Address	12 Wooburn Green, Russell Square, London
Social and family history	Teacher
	Lives with two children, aged 4 and 7, and her partner of 18 months
Past medical history	Gestational diabetes
Current medication	Nil
Note	Patient has bruises around her neck

BRAINSTORM

INSTRUCTIONS TO ROLE PLAYER (PATIENT OR CARER)

You are Sarah Fountain, a maths teacher.

You come to see the doctor because your eldest child has started to wet the bed.

Your husband left you while you were pregnant with your second child.

Your partner of 18 months has hit you many times in front of the children. You don't admit this straight away but you have bruises on your neck that the doctor should enquire about.

You eventually explain that the bruises were caused by him strangling you, and also admit that he's hit the children.

Opening statement:

'Hello doctor, Ellie, my eldest, has started to wet the bed.'

Freely divulged in response to open questions:

When the doctor asks for more detail, you hesitate and disclose that she's been doing this for 2 months.

You don't openly admit your domestic situation but look desperately sad and coy; you brush off the bruises around your neck as being caused by a fall.

Information divulged if asked specifically:

If pushed, you finally admit the bruises were due to Darren strangling you; he's punched you many times, usually after drinking; he's very controlling.

You're relieved that he's away on business for the next 10 days.

He threatened you when you wanted to leave in the past.

Again, if pushed, you admit that he has hit you in front of the children.

He has punched and kicked you several times; you have been in the emergency department with broken ribs in the past.

The neck bruising was caused by him strangling you.

Finally, you break down and admit that he smacked the children before he went away, and that was the final straw.

You're not depressed, or suicidal.

You admit that you need help and don't know what to do.

You're happy for social services to be contacted.

Your performance at work is slipping and you're happy to be signed off.

Your parents haven't spoken to you for many years.

You don't want to be examined by the doctor today.

CHAPTER 4

NOTES

OVERALL AIM OF THE CASE

To be able to pick up on cues to understand a hidden agenda, manage a very sensitive issue with safeguarding in mind, and offer reassurance and hope.

DATA GATHERING, TECHNICAL AND ASSESSMENT SKILLS

- It is important to explore why Ellie has started to wet herself.

- Two months of bedwetting is unlikely to be related to an infection, although there may be medical causes. It is the domestic situation that is the most likely culprit.

- It is useful to obtain the social background, support structure and history of how her partner has assaulted her and the children.

- Obtain her views on the GP contacting social services. What concerns does she have?

CLINICAL MANAGEMENT SKILLS

- This is a safeguarding issue for both the patient and her children.

- A referral to social services is entirely appropriate.

- Ellie should be reviewed to exclude a medical cause for her bedwetting, but this may need to be performed by a police surgeon or designated paediatric consultant.

INTERPERSONAL SKILLS

- The patient offers obvious cues; without picking up on these, you may not get to her hidden agenda.

CHAPTER 4

- This is a very emotive and sensitive subject and needs to be handled with appropriate tact.

- She needs to be enabled to express herself without embarrassment.

- Use silence to draw out important but deep emotions or sensitive information.

- Deal with her emotions with care and professionalism.

- Offer hope and support.

KEY POINTS

- Domestic abuse affects one in four women and one in six men.

- Abuse tends to increase during pregnancy.

- Women are subjected to 37 episodes of violence on average before seeking help.

- Domestic abuse (adults and children) is high on the agenda.

- Referral processes need to be streamlined and education and training improved.

- Effective multi-agency working is currently a challenge and must be improved.

- Out-of-hours provision of care is recognised as a challenge.

- Robust information sharing is a key objective.

FURTHER READING

British Medical Association. *The role of health professionals in identifying and responding to domestic abuse, including child and elder abuse.* London: BMA, 2011. Available at: bma.org.uk/working-for-change/improving-and-protecting-health/healthcare-for-vulnerable-groups/domestic-abuse.

CHAPTER 4

CASE 10

IN THIS STATION ...

You are the duty GP at the practice.

MATERIALS AND INSTRUCTIONS TO CANDIDATE (CASE NOTES)

Name	Patrick Van Der Bürg
Age	39 years
Address	90 The Pastures, Kentish Town, London NW5
Social and family history	Manager, printing firm
	Lives with mother
	Mother is on warfarin for recurrent DVTs (deep vein thromboses)
Past medical history	Mitral valve prolapse
	OA (osteoarthritis) of the knees
	Obesity
	Spontaneous DVT
Current medication	Paracetamol
Previous consultation (last week)	Calf pain, left, 5 days, painful
	o/e afebrile, pitting oedema, red, tender, Well's DVT score: high
	Can't exclude DVT, refer
Hospital report	D-dimer 3426 ng/ml
	CRP (C-reactive protein) 3 mg/dl
Ultrasound report	'No evidence of thrombosis or Baker's cyst seen. No groin lymphadenopathy'

CHAPTER 4

BRAINSTORM

EXAMINATION FINDINGS
Information offered on iPad if appropriate

Afebrile

Whole left leg swollen

Calf circumference 5 cm greater than right leg

Dilated (non-varicose) superficial left leg veins

Tender along distribution of deep left leg veins

INSTRUCTIONS TO ROLE PLAYER (PATIENT OR CARER)

You are Patrick Van Der Bürg, a printer.

You were referred for a possible DVT last week.

Your blood test was highly suggestive of a DVT at the clinic but the scan was negative for a thrombosis.

Your leg seems to be getting worse; the whole leg is now affected.

Opening statement:

'Hi doctor, I'm really worried about my leg ... .'

Freely divulged in response to open questions:

You explain that you're worried that the leg getting worse.

It's getting more painful and swollen; the whole leg is now affected.

Information divulged if asked specifically:

You have no idea what is causing your symptoms given that the scan was clear.

It feels exactly the same as the last time you had a DVT.

You don't understand why you need a repeat scan if the ultrasound scan last week was normal.

You know that DVTs can cause an embolus.

You wonder if you and your mum share a genetic condition and you've not been tested for this.

You've been physically active and have not had any periods of immobility; you've not travelled in the last 6 months.

You've never smoked.

You feel well otherwise.

You don't feel feverish.

CHAPTER 4

NOTES

OVERALL AIM OF THE CASE

To have the courage of your convictions, despite the hospital apparently excluding a diagnosis.

DATA GATHERING, TECHNICAL AND ASSESSMENT SKILLS

- The differential diagnosis of a swollen leg in this case is either an infection or a missed DVT.

- The whole leg is affected and, given the ultrasound report, a Baker's cyst is unlikely

- It's important to appreciate that the CRP is an acute phase protein; the fact that it is normal makes an infection unlikely.

- It is worth exploring information about his mother's condition.

CLINICAL MANAGEMENT SKILLS

- Despite a normal ultrasound scan last week, given the clinical findings it is very reasonable to re-refer the patient and ask the DVT clinic to make a further assessment.

- Antibiotics would not be appropriate.

INTERPERSONAL SKILLS

- This case requires an explanation to the patient of how no test is perfect and persuading him that a repeat scan may be useful.

- Checking the patient's understanding is appropriate, particularly about what a DVT is.

- Ensuring that the patient knows what to expect, eg a repeat blood test and scan, and potentially warfarin will reduce his anxiety.

KEY POINTS

- Venous thromboembolic disease accounts for 10 times more deaths than MRSA (meticillin-resistant *Staphylococcus aureus*) infection.

- Patients with proximal DVTs (thigh and pelvic venous disease) are most at risk of severe complications and death.

- Some data suggest that superficial vein thrombosis is a marker for DVT in 5% of cases

- D-dimer has a high negative predictive value for DVTs.

- A false positive D-dimer can occur in the presence of rheumatoid factor.

CHAPTER 4

CASE 11

IN THIS STATION ...

You are a GP in the practice.

MATERIALS AND INSTRUCTIONS TO CANDIDATE (CASE NOTES)

Name	Brenda Andrews
Age	75 years
Address	Hulfords House, Montague Square, London W1
Social and family history	Lives with husband, who has dementia
Past medical history	Hypertension
	Cervical spondylosis
	GORD (gastro-oesophageal reflux disease)
	CKD (chronic kidney disease) stage 3
	Obesity
Current medication	Amlodipine 5 mg od
	Ramipril 2.5 mg od
	Omeprazole 20 mg od
	Paracetamol 1000 mg max qds
Previous consultation (2 weeks ago – telephone)	Patient reviewed for SOBOE
	Full blood count (FBC), CXR (chest X-ray) and spirometry normal
	Plan: open access echo and review in clinic

Echocardiography report	Structurally normal valves
	Normal systolic function
	Grade II diastolic dysfunction
	Mild concentric LVH (left ventricular hypertrophy)
Conclusion	Diastolic heart failure, hypertensive heart disease; advise improving blood pressure control

CHAPTER 4

BRAINSTORM

EXAMINATION FINDINGS
Information offered on iPad if appropriate

Sinus rhythm 90 beats/min

BP 168/92 mmHg, 174/96 mmHg and 168/94 mmHg

BMI (body mass index) 35 kg/m^2

INSTRUCTIONS TO ROLE PLAYER (PATIENT OR CARER)

You are Brenda Andrews.

You have a long history of high blood pressure; you're embarrassed to admit that you often don't take your amlodipine because it causes ankle swelling.

You've been experiencing breathlessness on exertion for a year, which is slowly getting worse.

You've had several tests that have come back clear. You've come to get the results of your heart scan.

Opening statement:

'Morning doctor, I've come to get my results.'

Freely divulged in response to open questions:

You've been breathless for around a year.

You've seen another GP who checked that you weren't anaemic; he also organised a chest X-ray and blow tests, and said that your lungs were perfect.

You then spoke to a doctor on the phone who said that the next step was a heart scan.

Information divulged if asked specifically:

You don't know what the result of the scan showed, except to say that the echocardiographer said it wasn't normal; he used some technical terms but you didn't understand them.

You are not sure why you had a heart scan; you thought breathlessness was due to lung disease.

You never get chest pain. You've never smoked.

You eventually admit to not taking your amlodipine regularly because it makes your ankles swell; you have several boxes at home.

You had no idea high blood pressure can make the heart 'thick' and stiff. You find the term 'diastolic heart failure' frightening.

You only get breathless when you walk quickly or up a hill, never at rest.

The breathing doesn't stop you looking after your husband but you do feel that he is deteriorating with his dementia.

You agree to the doctor's medical plan.

CHAPTER 4

NOTES

OVERALL AIM OF THE CASE

To articulate a complicated result and manage the patient's expectations.

DATA GATHERING, TECHNICAL AND ASSESSMENT SKILLS

- Establish the history so far.
- Checking patients are taking their drugs as prescribed is critical. If not, why not?
- How is the breathlessness affecting her life?
- Establish whether there are any associated cardiac symptoms.
- Is she coping with her husband having dementia?
- The pulse and blood pressure should be checked.

CLINICAL MANAGEMENT SKILLS

- Substituting amlodipine for a drug that slows the heart down (allowing the heart greater filling time) would be a reasonable next step; this would also resolve her concern about ankle swelling.
- Diuretics may be considered.
- It is important to manage the blood pressure to ensure that it is consistently well controlled.
- Offer to organise a home visit to discuss her husband's situation.

INTERPERSONAL SKILLS

- Does the patient understand why heart problems can cause breathlessness?

- Explaining what diastolic heart failure means in appropriate language is essential.

- Recognise that the word 'failure' can be emotive.

- Managing the patient's expectations is important; her breathlessness may not improve at all with the new regimen.

KEY POINTS

- Failure of the heart muscle to relax is a useful way to think about diastolic dysfunction.

- It is more common in women.

- Risk factors include high blood pressure, aortic stenosis, hypertrophic cardiomyopathy and amyloid.

- It may lead to atrial dilatation and atrial fibrillation.

- Heart rate and cardiac risk factors should be controlled; diuretics may be tried.

CHAPTER 4

CASE 12

IN THIS STATION ...

You are a new GP; you've been asked to do a home visit at the local day centre on one of your practice's patients.

MATERIALS AND INSTRUCTIONS TO CANDIDATE (CASE NOTES)

Name	Henry Parry
Age	86 years
Address	12 Drayton Drive, West Ealing, London
Social and family history	Lives with wife who has dementia
	Attends day centre three times a week
	Mobilises with an electric scooter
	Care package twice a day
Past medical history	Severe osteoarthritis
Current medication	Paracetamol 500 mg 2 qds
	Naproxen 250 mg prn
	MST 10 mg m/r bd

CHAPTER 4

BRAINSTORM

CHAPTER 4

EXAMINATION FINDINGS
Information offered on iPad if appropriate

Poorly animated facies

Resting tremor

Cogwheeling

Lead-pipe rigidity

Shuffling gait

Signs of generalised osteoarthritis

INSTRUCTIONS TO ROLE PLAYER (PATIENT OR CARER)

You are Henry Parry, a retired army officer who is currently at the local day centre.

You have severe arthritis in both knees after a training accident 50 years ago.

You mobilise with a scooter.

The staff have called the doctor to see you because they have noticed a tremor in your left hand.

Opening statement:

'Hello doctor, sorry to trouble you, I wouldn't have called but the girls here insisted.'

Freely divulged in response to open questions:

You've had the tremor in your left hand for at least 6 months and you've stopped driving as a consequence.

It's not bothered you that much. You've got more important things to worry about than the tremor (your arthritic pain and your wife who has dementia – you don't expand on this unless doctor asks).

Information divulged if asked specifically:

You're left handed.

The tremor usually occurs when you're not moving your hand; your arm feels very stiff and it's difficult to move it quickly.

You can walk at home (a ground floor adapted flat) with a frame.

Your knees are very painful; you can't face having a knee replacement. You can't take big steps anymore – you can't help but shuffle along. You haven't fallen.

Thinking about it, your tremor is affecting you a lot and you play it down. You can barely write and you can't cook anymore. Washing and dressing are very difficult now.

Some people say that you stare and your facial movements seem slow.

Your wife has dementia and you know that she needs to go to a nursing home, especially as you can't look after her. You feel very guilty.

You're not depressed, and life is worth living but you are worried about the future.

Your only child is in the army and can't help you.

You're worried about Parkinson's disease and would be happy to be referred to a neurologist and to have more care at home.

NOTES

OVERALL AIM OF THE CASE

To introduce the idea of a life-changing illness and putting it into the patient's social context.

DATA GATHERING, TECHNICAL AND ASSESSMENT SKILLS

- The data gathering ought to be split into logical sections, perhaps summarising after each one to ensure that you understand the patient and the patient understands you.

- It is reasonable to enquire about the nature of the tremor, how well he can function at home and his mental health.

- Basic questions about the tremor and associated features point towards a diagnosis of Parkinson's disease

- Performing a directed examination will reveal signs of Parkinson's disease

- Enquiring about how he is managing at home, whether his care package is adequate, his arthritis and how he manages looking after his wife are all important issues.

CLINICAL MANAGEMENT SKILLS

- A referral to a neurologist to confirm Parkinson's disease and start treatment can improve his functioning and ensure that he is put in touch with the relevant support networks.

- Social services referral is needed to ensure that he and his wife are looked after; this may entail increasing the care package and/or sourcing alternative living arrangements.

CHAPTER 4

INTERPERSONAL SKILLS

- Establish what the patient's views are on a referral to neurology and the care-of-the-elderly team.

- Sharing options and discussing possible solutions with the patient will empower him and make him feel valued.

- Enquiring about his functioning in a supportive way will demonstrate a real commitment to help.

KEY POINTS

- Parkinsonism may be caused by drugs, stroke and tumours as well as Parkinson's disease

- Parkinson's disease is the most common neurodegenerative disease and the incidence increases with age.

- Smoking appears to be protective.

- Key features of Parkinson's disease are resting tremor, lead-pipe rigidity, akinesia/bradykinesia and postural instability.

- The symptoms are usually asymmetrical and affect the arms more than the legs.

- Difficulty smelling, constipation and sleep disorder may represent a prodrome to Parkinson's disease.

- Treatment is complicated and includes drug therapy and possible neurosurgery.

- A multidisciplinary team (MDT approach) is important, including GP, neurologist, specialist nurses, physiotherapists, occupational therapists and neuropsychiatrists.

FURTHER READING

For a comprehensive review of Parkinson's disease: www.gponline.com/ Clinical/article/986869/Clinical-Review---Parkinson's-disease.

Parkinson's disease Society: www.parkinsons.org.uk.

CHAPTER 4

CASE 13

IN THIS STATION ...

You are a new GP at the practice.

MATERIALS AND INSTRUCTIONS TO CANDIDATE (CASE NOTES)

Name	Dilip Patel
Age	40 years
Address	42a New Road, Kings Cross, London
Social and family history	Grocer
	Lives with wife and three children
	Smokes 20/day
Past medical history	Nil
Current medication	Nil

CHAPTER 4

BRAINSTORM

EXAMINATION FINDINGS
Information offered on iPad if appropriate

No cachexia

No pallor/jaundice

Abdomen looks normal

Generally tender epigastrium

No discrete masses

No organomegaly

No ascites detected

CHAPTER 4

INSTRUCTIONS TO ROLE PLAYER (PATIENT OR CARER)

You are Dilip Patel, a London grocer.

You work hard and long hours.

You've been complaining of abdominal pain for 8 weeks.

Opening statement

'Hello doctor, thanks for seeing me, I've got tummy pain.'

Freely divulged in response to open questions:

The pain is here (you point to the area above your belly button [epigastrium for the medically minded]).

It hurts almost all the time.

Information divulged if asked specifically:

The pain is a dull fire-like pain.

The pain doesn't spread anywhere.

You have no difficulties in swallowing.

You've not lost weight.

You've not vomited.

You've not lost your appetite.

You take over-the-counter aspirin as you think this will stop you getting a heart attack.

Your blood group is B positive.

There are no stomach problems in your or your family's history.

Your bowel habit is normal and your stool is neither black nor bloody.

NOTES

OVERALL AIM OF THE CASE

To manage a common complaint and to exclude sinister pathology.

DATA GATHERING, TECHNICAL AND ASSESSMENT SKILLS

- As with all pains, it should be explored in detail. This will include location, nature, consistency, onset, triggers, exacerbating and relieving factors, radiation, timing and associated features.

- In addition, red flags should be explored and excluded or acted upon.

- A competent gastrointestinal examination may be required in the CSA examination

CLINICAL MANAGEMENT SKILLS

- The aspirin should be stopped.

- The patient should be referred for *Helicobacter pylori* breath testing (many practices perform tests) and a PPI (proton pump inhibitor) commenced as soon as the test has been completed.

- Smoking cessation advice.

- Safety netting and appropriate follow-up to discuss the *H. pylori* results.

INTERPERSONAL SKILLS

- Use language that the patient understands.

- Consider what the patient's thoughts are on the condition and why he thinks that he has it.

- What are his views on smoking: does he want to give up? If not, does he understand the risks?

CHAPTER 4

119

KEY POINTS

Urgent referral for suspect cancer (NICE *Referral guidelines for suspected cancer*, 2005):

- Dysphagia at any age abdominal mass or obstructive jaundice.

- Dyspepsia at any age combined with one or more of the following:

  - Weight loss

  - Proven anaemia (iron deficiency)

  - Vomiting (persistent)

  - Dysphagia

  - Chronic GI bleeding

  - Weight loss

  - Epigastric mass.

- Dyspepsia in a patient aged ≥55 years with at least one of the following:

  - Onset of dyspepsia <1 year ago

  - Continuous symptoms since onset.

- Dyspepsia combined with at least one of the following known risk factors:

  - Family history of upper gastrointestinal (GI) cancer in more than two first-degree relatives

  - Barrett's oesophagus

  - Pernicious anaemia

  - Peptic ulcer surgery >20 years before

  - Known dysplasia, atrophic gastritis or intestinal metaplasia.

CHAPTER 4

120

BONUS CASE

IN THIS STATION …

You are a new GP at the practice.

MATERIALS AND INSTRUCTIONS TO CANDIDATE (CASE NOTES)

Name	Fran Taylor
Age	80 years
Address	52a Hollies Road, Charing Cross, London
Social and family history	Lives with daughter, Nancy
Past medical history	AF
	TIA
	Hypertension
Current medication	Aspirin 75 mg od
	Digoxin 125 mcg od
	Bisoprolol 5 mg od

Medication review overdue

BRAINSTORM

EXAMINATION FINDINGS

Information offered on iPad if appropriate

Ventricular rate 76 beats/min

BP 134/70 mmHg

HS (heart sounds) normal

INSTRUCTIONS TO ROLE PLAYER (PATIENT OR CARER)

You are Fran Taylor, a retired nurse.

You have come to get a medication review. The doctor will persuade you to take warfarin rather than aspirin; you are initially resistant but will be persuaded by good arguments.

Opening statement:

'Hello doctor, I've only come in for my medication review.'

Freely divulged in response to open questions:

You feel well.

You don't have any concerns about your health.

You'd like to cut down on your medications if possible.

Information divulged if asked specifically:

You don't experience breathlessness, chest pain, palpitations or dizziness.

You don't really understand what AF is.

You don't know why people make such a fuss of it.

You don't understand why you can't just take aspirin to reduce your stroke risk.

You believe aspirin is much safer than warfarin.

You don't want new generation drugs to thin the blood because you don't believe that they are tried and tested.

CHAPTER 4

NOTES

OVERALL AIM OF THE CASE

To use the CHADS2 score to establish a patient requires anticoagulation and to persuade her of the benefits.

DATA GATHERING, TECHNICAL AND ASSESSMENT SKILLS

- To understand the patient's symptoms and current cardiovascular status.

- This includes the ventricular rate and manual blood pressure given that automated machines are not always accurate in AF.

- To perform the CHADS2 score (4 in this case) and recognise that this requires anticoagulation.

CLINICAL MANAGEMENT SKILLS

- Refer for initiation of anticoagulation

- Follow-up.

INTERPERSONAL SKILLS

- To explain in simple language what AF is and why it is so important to manage properly.

- To translate the evidence in simple language that aspirin performs poorly against warfarin in stroke risk reduction.

CHAPTER 4

KEY POINTS

- AF is common because 30% of patients are asymptomatic.

- AF is increasing in prevalence over time.

- The risk of stroke is increased fivefold in AF (and paroxysmal AF).

- All-cause mortality is higher with AF compared with sinus rhythm, especially in women.

- Stroke outcomes are worse in AF compared with those in sinus rhythm; the chances of independent living are reduced, and depression and quality of life are worse in AF.

- Aspirin is an anti-platelet agent whereas clot in AF is fibrin rich, which responds better to warfarin.

- Warfarin is superior in stroke risk reduction than aspirin alone or aspirin combined with clopidogrel.

- Aspirin is no safer than warfarin and is less effective with age in stroke risk reduction in AF.

- The $CHADS_2$ score has been superseded by the CHA_2DS_2-VASc score but has been included here as $CHADS_2$ is currently adopted by QOF.

CHAPTER 4

Chapter 5
Exam Circuit 2

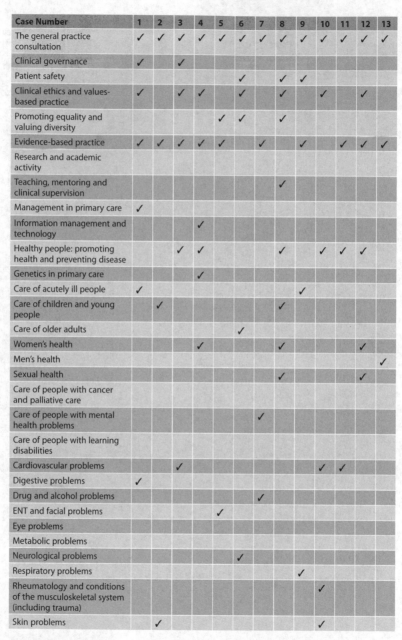

Case Number	1	2	3	4	5	6	7	8	9	10	11	12	13
The general practice consultation	✓	✓	✓	✓	✓	✓	✓	✓	✓	✓	✓	✓	✓
Clinical governance	✓		✓										
Patient safety						✓		✓	✓				
Clinical ethics and values-based practice	✓		✓	✓		✓		✓		✓		✓	
Promoting equality and valuing diversity					✓	✓		✓					
Evidence-based practice	✓	✓	✓	✓	✓		✓		✓		✓	✓	✓
Research and academic activity													
Teaching, mentoring and clinical supervision								✓					
Management in primary care	✓												
Information management and technology			✓										
Healthy people: promoting health and preventing disease			✓	✓				✓		✓	✓	✓	
Genetics in primary care			✓										
Care of acutely ill people	✓								✓				
Care of children and young people		✓						✓					
Care of older adults						✓							
Women's health				✓				✓				✓	
Men's health													✓
Sexual health								✓				✓	
Care of people with cancer and palliative care													
Care of people with mental health problems							✓						
Care of people with learning disabilities													
Cardiovascular problems			✓							✓	✓		
Digestive problems	✓												
Drug and alcohol problems							✓						
ENT and facial problems				✓									
Eye problems													
Metabolic problems													
Neurological problems						✓							
Respiratory problems									✓				
Rheumatology and conditions of the musculoskeletal system (including trauma)											✓		
Skin problems		✓								✓			

Fig. 4 Circuit 2 cases plotted against RCGP curriculum

CASE 1

INSTRUCTIONS TO THE CANDIDATE (CASE NOTES)

You are a locum GP and have never worked in the practice before.

Name	Matthew Johnson
Age	74 years
Address	92a Rycknield Street, Woodburn Green, HP10 9LL
Social and family history	Lives with wife
Past medical history	COPD
	Angina
	Hypertension
	Cancer of the bowel, 2009, resected with end-to end anastomosis
Current medication	Salbutamol – PRN
	Tiotropium – one puff daily
	Aspirin 75 mg od
	Atenolol 50 mg od
	Ramipril 10 mg od
	Simvastatin 40 mg nocte
	Isosorbide mononitrate 10 mg bd
Additional info (results/letters)	ALERTS: medication review overdue
	Colorectal department summary letter dated 2011 (enclosed)

CHAPTER 5

> Wycombe Hospital
> High Wycombe
> Buckinghamshire
> HP11 2PT

12 Grange Road,
High Wycombe
6/12/2011

Dear Mr Johnson

I am delighted to report that the biopsy results from your recent colonoscopy are benign and show no signs of residual cancer following your recent operation. We will send you an appointment for a follow-up colonoscopy in about 6 months' time.

Yours sincerely

Mr Bason

Consultant colorectal surgeon

MBBS, FRCS (London)

BRAINSTORM

INSTRUCTIONS TO THE ROLE PLAYER (PATIENT)

NOT TO BE SEEN BY THE CANDIDATE

Patient background:

You are 74-year-old Matthew Johnson. You are a retired printer.

You have come for a medication review having received a couple of recent letters inviting you for this. You take a variety of tablets and puffers, and you think that some are for your lungs and some for your heart.

You would like loperamide added to your regular medicines because you have been using this to control your loose motions in the last few months.

You want to take the opportunity to ask the doctor why you never had any follow-up after your bowel cancer as had been implied when you last saw the colorectal specialist a few years ago. You had not been bothered about this until now because you have had fresh blood mixed with your stools for a couple of months and are worried that the cancer may have recurred; this is how the concern first presented.

You feel a bit stupid for not having asked about the lack of follow-up before now. You moved house shortly after your bowel operation and suspect that any letters from the hospital may have gone to your old address.

You decline an examination if offered but accept a referral back to the surgeons. You are not angry at the practice but would like to know if there has been a mistake.

Opening statement:

'I've come so that you can check my medicines.'

Freely divulged in response to open questions:

Sorry that it's taken so long to come in.

You would like loperamide added to regular script as you've been needing a lot for last few months.

Information divulged if asked specifically:

You think that the cancer is back.

You think that there has been an oversight in not having been contacted for follow-up.

Worried because 2 months of fresh PR bleeding and 3 months of change to loose motions.

No abdominal pain, fever, weight loss, bone pain.

No anal symptoms to suggest piles/fissure.

No family history of bowel/related cancers.

Feel guilty and stupid because you did not chase the colorectal follow-up before now.

NOTES

OVERALL AIM OF THE CASE

Identifying the patient's hidden agenda for coming and recognising red flags for colorectal cancer.

Appreciating the significant error that has occurred with regard to the lack of follow-up after the bowel resection.

DATA GATHERING, TECHNICAL AND ASSESSMENT SKILLS

- Ensuring that you ask about ideas, concerns and expectations (ICE) will identify the patient agenda, ie colorectal symptoms.

- Colorectal history should include questions about family history of bowel cancer, and red flag symptoms that pertain to the 2WW referral criteria, ie change in bowel habit, absence of anal symptoms.

- Clarify address changes to ascertain how this loss of follow-up occurred and to prevent repetition.

- Offer examination including abdomen, digital rectal examination, BP, heart rate and checking for eyelid pallor.

CLINICAL MANAGEMENT SKILLS

- 2WW colorectal referral.

- In this instance the patient will be acquainted with colonoscopy having had it before, but offering an explanation in lay terms of what the patient can expect when they see the colorectal team will enhance a shared understanding of the plan.

- Offer support in the future, eg patient can call at any time with any concerns.

- Check addresses and ensure up to date on the practice system.

CHAPTER 5

- Significant event analysis (SEA). Suggest to the patient that you will bring this event to the attention of the practice team who will look at how and why he got left to follow-up.

- If the patient wants to make a formal complaint demonstrate knowledge of how this process works, ie written letter delivered to the practice manager who would respond within a prescribed time frame.

- Good medical practice specifies that you must respect the skills and contributions of your colleagues, ie do not be tempted to criticise colleagues even if a patient tries to draw you into this.

- ± medication review, although this is not a priority.

INTERPERSONAL SKILLS

- Allow the patient to express his thoughts about what happened without interruption

- Use active listening skills, eg verbal and non-verbal signals

- Express empathy for the patient's situation

- Apologise for systematic mistake.

FURTHER READING

NICE. *Referral guidelines for suspected cancer*, 2005. www.nice.org.uk/guidance/CG27

NICE have produced clear guidance on 'urgent' referral under the 2 week wait rule for different suspected types of cancer. Criteria for urgent referral of suspected lower GI cancer are as follows:

- All ages: definite, palpable, right-sided abdominal mass consistent with involvement of the large bowel, definite, palpable rectal (intraluminal, not pelvic) mass, unexplained iron deficiency anaemia (men <11 g/dl, non-menstruating women <10 g/dl)

- Age >40 years: rectal bleeding WITH a change of bowel habit to looser stools AND/OR increased frequency of defecation persisting for 6 or more weeks

CHAPTER 5

- Age >60 years: rectal bleeding without anal symptoms persisting for 6 or more weeks, change in bowel habit to looser motions persisting for 6 or more weeks

- In patients aged 60 years, *without* rectal bleeding, but a change in bowel habit to looser stools and/or more frequent stools persisting for 6 weeks (note that local guidelines may vary)

- In patients with equivocal symptoms, a full blood count can identify the possibility of colorectal cancers by demonstrating iron deficiency anaemia.

NHS bowel cancer screening programme (NHS BCSP). www.cancerscreening.nhs.uk/bowel/bowel-ipc-booklet.pdf

Programme rolled out nationally following pilots in four countries including the UK, which suggested that screening using faecal occult blood (FOB) might be viable within the context of the NHS. With a couple of exceptions, all people aged 60–69 in England have been sent an invitation letter to participate in screening. The uptake in the first phase was 59 per cent of respondents accepting the offer of testing and returning an FOB sample for analysis. The screening programme summary for GPs outlines the algorithm for individuals, depending on their FOB sample result. In the first phase, 16 of 1000 FOB results showed a positive result. These individuals are offered a meeting with a specialist nurse within a week of receiving their positive FOB result, and are assessed to see if colonoscopy is appropriate. In the first phase, 78 per cent of individuals offered colonoscopy accepted this procedure. Ten per cent of those who underwent colonoscopy were diagnosed as having colorectal cancer.

CASE 2

INSTRUCTIONS TO THE CANDIDATE (CASE NOTES)

Name	Fiona McQuirk
Age	16 years
Address	101 Shortbutts Lane, High Wycombe
Social and family history	Non-smoker
Past medical history	Acne vulgaris
Current medication	Clindamycin/benzoyl peroxide gel daily (Duac)
	Azelaic acid ointment
Additional info (results/letters)	Nil

BRAINSTORM

INSTRUCTIONS TO THE ROLE PLAYER (PATIENT)

NOT TO BE SEEN BY THE CANDIDATE

Patient background:

You are 16-year-old Fiona McQuirk. You have non-scarring acne affecting your face, neck, upper back and chest. You feel that a couple of prescribed topical gel treatments have not worked. You believe that poor hygiene underpins acne, and so washing must help.

You have read about retinoids online and have tried to obtain them on the internet without success. You know that you need a dermatology referral for oral retinoids and want your GP to arrange this straight away because you think that this is where your answer lies.

You get teased at school to the point where you have lost a lot of confidence. Your boyfriend teases you about your spotty chest. Partly because of this, you have not yet started having sex as you are embarrassed about your appearance.

Your mood is low but not suicidal.

YOU WILL NOT BE EXAMINED, AND IF THE CANDIDATE OFFERS AN EXAMINATION HE OR SHE WILL BE PASSED A PIECE OF PAPER WITH THE EXAMINATION FINDINGS BY THE EXAMINER.

Opening statement:

'The gels for my spots haven't worked. If anything, things are even worse. I want to see a skin specialist.'

Freely divulged in response to open questions:

Fed up with nothing working.

Wash face at least 10 times a day.

Hate school and can't wait to leave at the end of the year.

Even your boyfriend teases you about your spots.

Information divulged if asked specifically:

Tried clindamycin/benzoyl peroxide combination and azelaic acid.

Not tried topical retinoids or oral antibiotics.

Never been on the pill/Dianette.

Believe that oral retinoids would solve the problem.

Not having the intimate relationship that you desire with your boyfriend because too embarrassed about appearance.

Have not started having sex.

No contraindications to COC.

Attended today because efforts to obtain retinoids online have failed.

Regular periods

No excess hair on your body

NOTES

OVERALL AIM OF THE CASE

Dealing with a patient's expectations and reaching a shared management plan.

Understanding the patient's health beliefs and how she experiences her acne.

Demonstrating sensitivity to a patient who is psychologically troubled by a superficially 'minor' complaint.

DATA GATHERING, TECHNICAL AND ASSESSMENT SKILLS

- Why attend today?
- When did acne start and has it changed with time?
- Does she have any symptoms to suggest PCOS or other causes of hyperandrogenism?
- Effects of previous treatments.
- Tried anything else, eg over-the-counter or herbal remedies?
- Taking other medicines, eg pharmacy-only prescription, steroids and phenytoin can worsen acne.
- Other body image problems?
- Mood assessment: important to assess the psychosocial status of the patient
- Sexually active?
- Contraception and contraindications if COC considered.
- Offer to examine skin; if anywhere other than face offer a chaperone.
- What does she know about retinoids?
- Does she know that retinoid gels can be prescribed by a GP?

CHAPTER 5

CLINICAL MANAGEMENT SKILLS

- Provide the patient with options to demonstrate a flexible approach and allow the patient to 'own' the shared management plan.

- Ensure that the selection of therapy fits, and is suitable and acceptable to the patient's lifestyle.

- Options include topical retinoids, oral antibiotics, topical antibiotics, Dianette, dermatology referral, combination therapy if considering oral retinoids.

- Contraception if uses topical or oral retinoids.

- NICE recommend two trials of oral antibiotics before referral to specialist, but psychological distress could circumnavigate this requirement.

- If referring to a dermatologist arrange FBC, lipids and LFTs, and ensure that two forms of contraception offered to all women of childbearing age, if considering oral retinoid treatment.

- Dianette reserved for women with 'severe' acne who have not responded to oral antibiotics, or for severe hirsuitism. It is no longer licensed for contraception in the UK.

- Patients should be advised about the relative increased risk of venous thromboembolism with the use of dianette.

- Offer regular follow-up.

The discussion should emphasise that acne is a chronic disease. Long-term therapy is required. It is a slow-responding disorder, and there is a need for continued adherence to treatment.

INTERPERSONAL SKILLS

- Addressing the patient agenda

- Appreciating the psychological dimension of this diagnosis

- Explore patient's perception of the severity of her acne, eg no evidence that chocolate adversely affects acne

- Health beliefs: washing, diet, etc.

- Explore impact on life: school, social life, love life.

CHAPTER 5

FURTHER READING

NICE 2001 referral advice

www.nice.org.uk

NICE produce guidelines on referral criteria from primary care, for a number of common pathologies including acne vulgaris. In brief, NICE recommends two trials oral antibiotics before referral to a dermatologist, but the patient's psychological distress can circumnavigate this requirement.

BNF section on acne

www.bnf.org

Outlines treatment options for mild, moderate and severe forms of acne vulgaris

gpnotebook summarises management in a stepwise approach very succinctly.

www.gpnotebook.co.uk

- Mild: topical benzoyl peroxidase/antibiotics (erythromycin, clindamycin, tetracycline)/retinoids/combinations of two of the three above/azelaic acid as alternative or add-on, especially useful to reduce 'flushing' and redness of acneified skin. Topical therapy should include a topical retinoid, however.

- Moderate: oral antibiotics (tetracyclines usually first line with erythromycin second line), COC/co-cyprindiol in women (treat early if inflammatory to prevent scarring). Oral antibiotics include: oxytetracycline, erythromycin, minocycline (not advocated as first- or second-line treatment), doxycycline, lymecycline, trimethoprim. There is a high incidence with regard to *Propionibacteria acnes* resistance; adding benzoyl peroxide would help. Note that definition of acne treatment is not only on a level of activity but also on the degree of grease production, psychosocial impact of disease and scarring.

- Severe/recalcitrant: oral isotretinoin.

British Association Dermatology guidelines and patient leaflets (for example, search 'acne')

www.bad.org.uk

Pictures online

www.dermnet.com

CHAPTER 5

CASE 3

INSTRUCTIONS TO THE CANDIDATE (CASE NOTES)

Name	David Butler
Age	50 years
Address	18 Quarry Hill, High Wycombe
Social and family history	Ex-smoker (gave up 20 years ago)
Past medical history	Chronic kidney disease stage 3
	Cheiropompholyx
	Vasectomy
Current medication	Nil
Additional info (results/letters)	
	10/09:
	eGFR 58 (57 in 2011)
	ACR 2.4
	U&Es
	Bone profile
	Hb normal ranges
	BP 132/78

BRAINSTORM

INSTRUCTIONS TO THE ROLE PLAYER (PATIENT)

NOT TO BE SEEN BY THE CANDIDATE

Patient background:

You are an ANGRY 50-year-old David Butler. You are angry because an insurance company has said that your medical records include a diagnosis of 'chronic kidney disease'.

You are in the process of a stressful re-mortgaging because your self-employed business has hit hard times. You had consented for the GP to disclose medical information to the insurance company and had stated that you did not need to see the report before your GP sent it to them.

You are angry that you have never been told that you have chronic kidney disease (CKD), and are anxious about what it means for your health.

You wanted to see your usual GP, Dr Spencer, so are even more frustrated at having to see a locum.

You will remain angry unless the GP allows you to vent your anger without confrontation and apologises for the way that you have been made to feel.

Opening statement:

ANGRY DEMEANOUR, DO NOT SIT DOWN UNTIL THIS IS POLITELY SUGGESTED, FEEL FREE TO AD-LIB FOR A GOOD MINUTE ON WHY AND HOW ANGRY YOU ARE!

Some suggested content

'You guys have got some explaining to do.'

'What's all this about me having severe kidney disease?'

'And I can't even get to see Dr Spencer, but have to see you.'

Freely divulged in response to open questions:

STILL VENTING ANGER

Never knowingly had a problem with kidneys, never been mentioned by GP.

Can't have been on records 5 years ago when you arranged original mortgage.

You're paying much higher premium because of this on records.

You wish that you had asked to see the forms before they were sent.

You're hoping that there's been a mistake, so that you can get the mortgage sorted quickly.

Information divulged if asked specifically:

No family history of renal disease.

Don't know what function the kidneys serve in the body.

Non-smoker and no other known cardiovascular risk factors.

You don't take NSAIDs.

You don't take any regular medicines.

Re-mortgage; self-employed builder, re-mortgaging to avoid insolvency.

Live with wife; children have left home.

CHAPTER 5

NOTES

OVERALL AIM OF THE CASE

Handling an angry patient.

The focus is on the interpersonal skills domain.

DATA GATHERING, TECHNICAL AND ASSESSMENT SKILLS

- Clarify exactly what the patient is angry about
- What does the patient want now?
- Check the patient's understanding of CKD
- Clarify the social and 're-mortgage' situation
- Clarify how the diagnosis was made
- Check past medical history including cardiovascular risk factors
- Family history
- Medication history.

CLINICAL MANAGEMENT SKILLS

- The patient may want to see his medical records; be aware of how a patient makes this request through the practice manager.
- The patient may want to make a formal complaint (verbal/in writing): be aware of how a patient does this, again through the practice manager, and the obligation of a practice to make a prompt response and discuss complaints as part of clinical governance.
- Provide options for follow-up if the patient feels that this is needed.
- Avoid passing judgement or criticising colleagues.
- As CKD is an independent cardiovascular risk factor, there may be a place for discussing lifestyle measures, including diet, exercise, smoking, alcohol.

CHAPTER 5

- Explain standard monitoring, ie 6-monthly blood, urine and BP check for stage 3 CKD.

INTERPERSONAL SKILLS

- Adopt a non-confrontational approach physically (stay seated) and verbally (use a quiet, slower voice to lower the tension)
- Allow the patient to speak and vent his anger
- Empathise and acknowledge his emotions
- While a patient should be listened to, a doctor should not have to endure verbal or physical assault.

KEY POINTS AND FURTHER READING

NICE. *Early identification and management of chronic kidney disease in adults in primary and secondary care.* London: NICE, 2008. www.nice.org.uk/guidance/CG73

CKD is a common independent cardiovascular risk factor that often coexists with diabetes, hypertension and other cardiovascular disease. An estimated 4–5 per cent of the adult population will have CKD stages 3–5. Treatment can delay the progression of CKD and reduce the risk of cardiovascular disease end-points such as myocardial infarction and stroke. Many people with advanced CKD can remain undiagnosed due to a lack of symptoms until late in the disease. To encourage earlier recognition of a treatable disease, NICE produced guidelines for diagnosis and management of CKD in primary care.

Screening with an estimated glomerular filtration rate (eGFR) and a urine ACR should be offered to people in the following categories:

- Diabetes, hypertension, ischaemic heart disease, chronic heart failure, peripheral vascular disease and cerebral vascular disease, structural renal tract disease, renal calculi or prostatic hypertrophy, multisystem diseases with potential kidney involvement such as systemic lupus erythematosus, family history of stage 5 CKD or hereditary kidney disease, and people who have an opportunistic detection of haematuria or proteinuria.

CHAPTER 5

Treatment with an angiotensin-converting enzyme inhibitor or angiotensin receptor blocker should be offered to the following groups:

- People who do not have diabetes: ACR >70 *or* ACR >30 (proteinuria) + BP >140/90 *or* ACR <30 + BP meets hypertensive thresholds according to NICE hypertensive guidelines

- People with diabetes: ACR >2.5 (men) *or* ACR >3.5 (women).

Referral to renal services should be considered in the following groups:

- Stage 4 and 5 CKD (with or without diabetes)

- ACR ≥70 mg/mmol unless due to diabetes and already treated

- ACR ≥30 mg/mmol + haematuria

- 'Rapidly' declining eGFR (>5 ml/min per 1.73 m^2 in 1 year, or >10 ml/min per 1.73 m^2 within 5 years)

- Hypertension that remains poorly controlled despite the use of at least four antihypertensive drugs at therapeutic doses

- People with, or suspected of having, rare or genetic causes of CKD

- Suspected renal artery stenosis.

When CKD was first introduced to the Quality Outcomes Framework (QOF), many renal services found themselves inundated with primary care referrals. Since that time, most renal services have produced their own more proscriptive local guidelines for referral. These invariably echo the recommendations above, with the caveat that stage 4 CKD need be referred only if the individual has an eGFR below the 3rd centile for age.

CKD gained prominence as a diagnosis in recent years when it was introduced into the QOF. Many doctors assert that the identification of large swathes of the elderly population with a kidney 'disease' that is often no more than a natural decline in renal function is ageist, stigmatising and a potential barrier to affordable health insurance for patients.

CHAPTER 5

CASE 4

INSTRUCTIONS TO THE CANDIDATE (CASE NOTES)

Name	Sonali Sudarshi
Age	38 years
Address	10 Bains Drive, High Wycombe
Social and family history	College lecturer
	Lives with husband and two daughters
Past medical history	Depression
	Menorrhagia
	Coeliac disease
Current medication	Nil
Additional info (results/letters)	Nil

BRAINSTORM

INSTRUCTIONS TO THE ROLE PLAYER (PATIENT)

NOT TO BE SEEN BY THE CANDIDATE

Patient background:

You are 38-year-old Sonali Sudarshi. You are an eloquent college lecturer who holds alternative medical therapies in high regard, and would like to know the doctor's opinion regarding therapies for prevention and treatment of breast cancer. This has been prompted by the recent identification of a high risk *BRCA-1* mutation in your family.

Your sister had breast cancer aged 35, she has a pathogenic *BRCA-1* mutation, and is considering a bilateral mastectomy.

Your mother died of ovarian cancer aged 50 and your 60-year-old aunt has just tested positive for the *BRCA-1* mutation and elected to have a prophylactic mastectomy and oophorectomy.

You are still assimilating this information, and are currently exploring your options. You currently think that mistletoe, aloe vera and essiac (North American Indian anti-cancer mix) are your best options and cannot bear the thought of a mastectomy.

You are scared at the thought of undergoing genetic testing and feel guilty towards your two young daughters because you feel that you have burdened them with your family history. You think that all women in your family have the pathogenic gene change and so it follows that you and your two daughters will get breast and/or ovarian cancer if you do not do something about it.

You attend with an internet printout on one/more of your herbal therapies to show the doctor in the hope that they will endorse herbal remedies as a panacea, although you suspect that the doctor will dismiss them out of hand.

INTERNET ARTICLE PROVIDED – TO SHOW DOCTOR.

Opening statement:

'I need to know what you think about mistletoe, aloe vera and essiac for breast cancer prevention.'

CHAPTER 5

Freely divulged in response to open questions:

Family history of cancer and recent genetic diagnosis in family.

Not sure what you want to do but inclined to try herbal remedies prophylactically.

Have read extensively and spoken to a trained Chinese medicine specialist.

Seems to be lots of evidence on the internet that supports use of these medicines.

Offer an article in support of one of the medicines as 'evidence'.

Information divulged if asked specifically:

You think that you definitely carry the high-risk *BRCA-1* mutation 'because all the women in our family get cancer'.

You think that your two daughters must have the mutation.

Mastectomy sounds scary, and as you might want more children you are uncertain about oophorectomy.

What screening is available for you and your daughters?

NOTES

OVERALL AIM OF THE CASE

Handle the 'expert' patient in a professional and honest manner, respecting someone's health beliefs, and reaching a shared management plan that aims to satisfy the patient agenda while acting safely.

DATA GATHERING, TECHNICAL AND ASSESSMENT SKILLS

- Cancer family history (pedigree)

- Where did family members have their diagnoses and genetic testing?

- Any current health concerns, especially regarding breast/ovary symptoms?

- Understanding of pathogenic gene changes and how they are inherited

- Understanding of implications for a woman or a man if they have such a gene change

- Medication history: contraception, herbal medicines

- Use of herbal/other complementary and alternative medicines.

CLINICAL MANAGEMENT SKILLS

- Show integrity and honesty if you lack knowledge of subjects, but always offer to get back to her once you have had a chance to find out more.

- Recognise a high-risk cancer family history and offer appropriate referral. Communicate the true prior probability of her and her daughters having the high-risk mutation, ie patient has a 50 per cent chance of having the gene change IF her mother had the mutation (which is likely), and about a 90 per cent lifetime chance of breast

CHAPTER 5

155

cancer and about a 45 per cent lifetime chance of ovarian cancer *if* she does have the *BRCA-1* gene change.

- Daughters don't definitely carry a mutation – prior risk about 25 per cent.

- Explain a woman's lifetime risk of breast and ovarian cancer, ie about 1 in 10 women will get breast cancer in their lifetime and about 1 in 90 women will get ovarian cancer regardless of whether they have a pathogenic gene change.

- About 5 per cent (1 in 20) of breast/ovary cancers will be attributable to a pathogenic gene.

- Empower the patient in her search for answers, eg by suggesting respected websites such as Cancer Research UK, or by providing patient information leaflets.

- Offer options – meet again once have found out more about herbal remedies/evidence base, support groups, screening, genetics referral, surgical referral.

INTERPERSONAL SKILLS

- Show respect for a person's health beliefs whatever your own opinions

- Explore her ideas about breast cancer genetics

- Explore her health beliefs in terms of causation and prevention

- Use lay language to communicate 'risk', 'genes' and 'mutations'

- Social aspects, such as to whom she has spoken about this, and has she discussed this with her daughters?

- Acknowledge the 'worry' that can be generated from this situation.

KEY POINTS AND FURTHER READING

NICE. *Familial breast cancer: Classification and care of people at risk of familial breast cancer and management of breast cancer and related risks in people with a family history of breast cancer*. London: NICE, 2013. http://guidance. nice.org.uk/CG164

Identifying significant family histories can be difficult, but it is impossible if you do not even ask about a family history of cancer!

The role of the primary care doctor is to provide psychological support and to assess an individual's cancer risk to enable appropriate and timely referral to secondary services if indicated.

Criteria for referral to clinical genetics cancer services, in the context of breast and ovary cancer are as follows:

- One first-degree relative (FDR = sibling, parent, child) with breast cancer aged <40 years at diagnosis

- One FDR + another FDR/second-degree relative (SDR) diagnosed with breast cancer at any age

- One male FDR with breast cancer

- One FDR/SDR with breast cancer + one FDR/SDR with ovarian cancer at any age

- Two FDRs, or one FDR and one SDR, diagnosed with breast cancer at any age

- Three FDRs or SDRs diagnosed with breast cancer at any age

- Note that bilateral breast cancer in a single relative counts as two separate cancers as if they occurred in two different individuals

- The guidelines do not emphasise that the Ashkenazi Jewish population (Jewish people with descent from the mediaeval Jews of the German Rhineland) have a disproportionate prevalence of certain recognised BRCA-1 + BRCA-2 pathogenic changes, and so most such families will meet criteria for referral at less stringent levels.

Be aware that there are several cancer-predisposing gene changes associated with breast cancer. BRCA-1 and BRCA-2 are the most common of those currently known. Pathogenic BRCA-1 changes confer increased risks of breast and ovarian cancer whereas BRCA-2 changes confer slightly lower risks of these cancers, but a higher risk of a number of other related cancers (pancreatic, fallopian, stomach, male breast and prostate).

Anyone meeting the criteria for referral to secondary/tertiary care has at least a moderately increased risk of carrying a pathogenic cancer gene

CHAPTER 5

157

change. Clinical geneticists will calculate an individual's and their other family members' risks of having a cancer-predisposing gene change. There are computer programs based on large population data that assist in these calculations. Genetic testing is now offered in specialist genetic clinics to a person with a relative who has a personal history of breast or ovarian cancer, if the relative's combined *BRCA-1* and *BRCA-2* mutation carrier probability is 10% or more. You can refer for genetic testing for *BRCA-1*, *BRCA-2* and *TP53* mutations within 4 weeks of diagnosis of breast cancer.

There is no accepted ovarian cancer screening programme because none has been shown to meet the 'Wilson criteria', which need to be fulfilled before a screening programme is deemed worthwhile. A number of large population-based studies have looked at whether different screening techniques, including CA125, combined with pelvic ultrasonography are feasible. In the UK, the largest of these looking at screening women in moderate- and high-risk cancer families is the UK Familial and Ovarian Cancer Screening Study (UKFOCCS). This study stopped recruiting entrants in 2006 and has interim reports to suggest that screening is not even worthwhile in higher-risk families. Studies looking at screening the general population for ovarian cancer have not yet been deemed worthwhile with current screening techniques.

Women at increased risk of breast cancer should be 'breast aware' in line with Department of Health advice for all women. The National Breast Screening Programme (NBSP) offers 3-yearly mammograms to women from age 47, and on request 3 yearly after age 70 years; by 2016 this will extend to 73. Given the notional success of the breast screening programme, it is perhaps surprising to many that debate continues about whether population mammographic screening is actually beneficial, with a number of studies coming out of Scandinavia in recent times that suggest the contrary (see Jørgensen et al).

Mammograms have reduced sensitivity in younger women because the denser breast tissue makes interpretation of images more difficult. MRI is currently offered as an alternative in younger women, but has low specificity for breast cancer and results in high false-positive results, meaning more unnecessary interventional diagnostic procedures such as fine-needle aspiration (FNA).

CHAPTER 5

Annual mammographic surveillance is offered to women aged between 40 and 49 years at moderate risk of breast cancer, between 40 and 59 years at high risk, and between 40 and 69 years with known *BRCA-1* or *BRCA-2* mutation.

MRI is offered annually to women in particular high-risk groups from age 30 years in known *BRCA* mutation carriers and those with significantly high-risk status, and from as young as 20 years in certain other rarer breast cancer-causing syndromes.

Risk-reducing surgery (mastectomy and/or oophorectomy) is appropriate for a small proportion of women who are from high-risk families and should be managed by a multidisciplinary team. Surgery reduces but does not entirely eradicate the risk of subsequent cancer.

Jørgensen KG, Zhal P-H, Gøtzsche PC. Breast cancer mortality in organised mammography screening in Denmark: comparative study. *BMJ* 2010; 340, c1241.

Ernst E, Pittler MH, Wider B. *The Desktop Guide to Complementary and Alternative Medicine: An Evidence-Based Approach.* Mosby 2006.

If you would like to read more about the evidence base behind complementary and alternative medicines, *The Desktop Guide to Complementary and Alternative Medicine* by Edzard Ernst is an excellent reference book.

CHAPTER 5

CASE 5

INSTRUCTIONS TO THE CANDIDATE (CASE NOTES)

Name	June Hutchinson
Age	40 years
Address	38 Darnford Lane, High Wycombe
Social and family history	Married
Past medical history	Psoriasis
	Bilateral sensorineural deafness
	Strabismus surgery
Current medication	Dovobet cream
	Cetraben emollient
Additional info (results/letters)	Nil

BRAINSTORM

EXAMINATION FINDINGS

Information offered on iPad if appropriate and given to the candidate if and when they have performed an examination of the patient's sore throat.

- 36.6°C
- Capillary refill time (CRT) <2 s
- RR 12/min
- Ears: normal tympanic membranes bilaterally
- Throat: pink, no tonsillar enlargement
- Neck: no cervical lymph node enlargement
- Chest: normal breath sounds all zones, heart sounds normal.

INSTRUCTIONS TO THE ROLE PLAYER (PATIENT)

NOT TO BE SEEN BY THE CANDIDATE

Patient background:

You are 40-year-old June Hutchinson. You have profound bilateral deafness and lip-read. You are attending with a 1-week history of viral URTI symptoms, are already getting better, but made the appointment a few days before when you thought that you needed an antibiotic.

You are happy to leave without an antibiotic if you are content with the doctor's explanation.

You will only 'hear' words the doctor says when they are looking at you and allowing you to lip-read.

THE CANDIDATE WILL BE ALLOWED TO PERFORM AN ENT EXAMINATION WITH YOUR CONSENT, BUT WOULD BE STOPPED BY THE EXAMINER AND TOLD THAT THE CHEST EXAMINATION IS NORMAL SHOULD HE OR SHE OFFER THIS EXAMINATION AS WELL. HE OR SHE WILL BE GIVEN A PIECE OF PAPER WITH THE 'EXAMINATION FINDINGS' AT THE END OF THE EXAMINATION.

Opening statement:

'I've had a sore throat for over a week, and this cough doesn't want to shift.'

Freely divulged in response to open questions:

1 week cough.

Sore throat.

Hot for a few days at the end of the week, but better now.

Paracetamol and linctuses don't seem to help.

Antibiotics have made things better in the past.

Information divulged if asked specifically:

You are improving.

Non-productive cough.

No meningism symptoms (no headache, light not hurting your eyes).

No past medical history tonsillitis/LRTI/respiratory disease.

No worries, in fact think it's getting better on its own now.

Half-expected not to get an antibiotic.

Housewife, so no sick note issues.

Deaf from early childhood, told due to a severe infection, used hearing aids for a couple of years, but of no use now, just lip-reading and signing, no family history of deafness.

NOTES

OVERALL AIM OF THE CASE

Communicating with the hearing-impaired patient while dealing with a common presentation.

Handling a patient who demands a certain course of action, in this instance the issuing of an antibiotic.

DATA GATHERING, TECHNICAL AND ASSESSMENT SKILLS

- URTI history
- Excluding meningism symptoms
- Past history of URTI problems
- Focused upper respiratory tract examination after gaining verbal consent
- ICE
- How has the illness affected work/home life?
- Why is she consulting now?

CLINICAL MANAGEMENT SKILLS

- Explain the likely diagnosis, natural history and suggestions for management.
- Address the patient's ideas, concerns and expectations.
- If the patient is especially demanding, a delayed script might be considered.
- If a patient insists on a certain course of action, such as the issuing of an antibiotic, attempt to explain the reasoning behind current best practice, eg antibiotics may only serve to increase resistance, risk side

CHAPTER 5

effects such as thrush and diarrhoea, and are unlikely to facilitate recovery.

- Safety net with explicit time frame if it gets worse or if problem persists.

INTERPERSONAL SKILLS

- Face the patient and talk at a slow/normal rate with normal volume, clear diction but without exaggeration of oral movements.

- Check understanding at regular intervals in a non-patronising manner.

- Acknowledging a patient's worries reduces the chance of conflict if she presents with demands for treatment.

- What are the patient's worries if an antibiotic is not issued?

KEY POINTS AND FURTHER READING

DDA 1995 (Disability Discrimination Act). www.legislation.gov.uk

The Disability Discrimination Act 1995 (c 50) is an Act of the Parliament of the UK which makes it unlawful to discriminate against people in respect of their disabilities in relation to employment, the provision of goods and services, education and transport.

Centor criteria

Centor RM, Witherspoon JM, Dalton HP, et al. The diagnosis of strep throat in adults in the emergency room. *Medical Decision Making* 1981;**1**:239–46.

The Centor criteria were developed to help diagnose group A streptococcal throat infections, and differentiate them from more common infections (mainly viral). The patients are judged on four criteria:

1. History of fever

2. Tonsillar exudates

3. Tender anterior cervical adenopathy

4. Absence of cough.

The presence of all four variables indicates a 40–60 per cent positive predictive value for a culture of the throat to test positive for group A streptococci. The absence of all four variables indicates a negative predictive value of greater than 80 per cent. The high negative predictive value suggests that the Centor criteria can be more effectively used for ruling out strep throat than for diagnosing strep throat.

NICE. *Respiratory Tract Infections – Antibiotic prescribing: prescribing of antibiotics for self-limiting respiratory tract infections in adults and children in primary care.* London: NICE, 2008. www.nice.org.uk/guidance/CG69.

These guidelines summarise an evidence-based approach to the common respiratory presentations. Cases are divided into those with and those without a high risk of complications. Specific presentations are dealt with in turn, with the common message being to consider not prescribing or using a delayed script preferentially. Presentations include acute otitis media, sore throat, acute pharyngitis, tonsillitis, common cold, acute rhinosinusitis and acute bronchitis. A doctor should also offer an idea of the expected natural history for these presentations.

The Faculty of Sexual and Reproductive Healthcare (FSRH) have advised that additional precautions are not required when using antibiotics.

FSRH. *CEU Combined Hormonal Contraception*, 2012. www.fsrh.org/pdfs/CEUGuidanceCombinedHormonalContraception.pdf

CHAPTER 5

CASE 6

INSTRUCTIONS TO THE CANDIDATE (CASE NOTES)

Name	Bernie Barnes
Age	60 years
Address	3 Waverley Walk, High Wycombe
Social and family history	Smoker 10/day
Past medical history	Hypertension
	Osteoarthritis
	Recurrent cystitis
Current medication	Bendroflumethiazide 2.5 mg
	Simvastatin 40 mg nocte
Results	BP 138/84

BRAINSTORM

INSTRUCTIONS TO THE ROLE PLAYER (PATIENT)

NOT TO BE SEEN BY THE CANDIDATE

(You are a third party and the GP will not have 'your' notes.)

Patient background:

You are 60-year-old Leonie Bell and are the long-term partner of Bernie. You are coming to see your partner's GP because you are worried about his memory loss.

You are not registered at the same practice and so the GP will not have your personal medical notes. You are a retired landscape architect.

You have several chronic health problems yourself and were recently diagnosed with metastatic breast cancer, for which you are receiving palliative treatment.

You are worried about Bernie's memory loss, which seems to have worsened dramatically over the last year, and are anxious that he will be left alone and unsupported when you die as he has no other family support.

You think that Bernie may have Alzheimer's disease, and were hoping that the GP would be able to see the patient without him knowing that you had approached in this way, to make an assessment, do tests and refer if necessary. You have heard that there are medicines for Alzheimer's disease.

You have a strained relationship with Bernie now, but do not feel that you could get out of the relationship if he has Alzheimer's disease, because you would feel too guilty to leave him if he needs your help.

Opening statement:

'I've come to talk about my partner Bernie. His memory's getting worse, and I think he has Alzheimer's.'

Freely divulged in response to open questioning:

Bernie has slowly deteriorated over several years.

His memory is appalling.

You can laugh about it sometimes but it's causing real problems now.

He is not the person you met 30 years ago.

He is often bad tempered these days.

Bernie does not know that you are seeing the GP and you don't want him to find out.

Divulged if asked specific questions:

'Appalling memory', eg forgot how to get back from shops and had to take taxi.

'Real problems', eg relationship breakdown; Bernie has expressed suicidal ideation without apparent intent.

'Bad tempered', eg started spitting at her, gets furious when he cannot remember where he has put things, not worried for personal safety.

Recent urine infection but treated and no problems now.

Bernie was an orphan and family history not known.

Bernie does not drive.

Bernie gave up smoking years ago – the records must be out of date.

NOTES

OVERALL AIM OF THE CASE

Recognise that in a 'third party' consultation you address the needs and agenda of the individual in front of you. Third party consultations require a working knowledge of the rules that underpin confidentiality, consent and working in a patient's best interests.

Demonstrate support for a patient's carer.

DATA GATHERING, TECHNICAL AND ASSESSMENT SKILLS

- Recognise that this is a third party consult.

- Does Bernie know that Leonie is here?

- Third party histories can be difficult but in the scenario presented, where the issue is memory loss, a clear history is essential.

- Why attending now?

- Why alone?

- Expectations of visit?

- What does Leonie know about dementia?

- History of Bernie's cognitive decline: when started, stepwise/gradual, associated features, diurnal variation, personality change, examples of changed behaviour, mood and suicidal risk, safety for Leonie (third party) and Bernie, clarify past medical history, signs of stroke/acute confusional state, medicine changes, unwell, ?UTI, impact on daily life.

- Does Bernie drive or work?

- Explore how you might arrange to meet with Bernie, ie would he come in to the surgery, home visit, send a letter inviting him for a general health check written in such a way as to make it seem like a routine appointment request?

- Does Bernie know that Leonie (third party) has a terminal diagnosis?

CLINICAL MANAGEMENT SKILLS

- Supporting Leonie (third party).

- Confidentiality: not sharing information from the clinical records with a third party.

- Consent: has Bernie given you, his GP, consent to approach him about this issue and, if not, what options might you explore with Leonie to get around this ethical obstacle, and would you be within your rights to approach him directly if you were 'acting in the patient's best interests'?

- Differential diagnosis explained.

- If Bernie consents, will happily see for assessment, and further investigations.

- Dementia diagnosis and management: psychogeriatricians, care packages, district nurses, carer support and respite, Age Concern, anticholinesterase medications.

INTERPERSONAL SKILLS

- The patient is primarily the person in front of you.

- Explain confidentiality issues as they apply to this case, ie although you can hear what Leonie has to say, you are confidentiality bound not to disclose information from the patient's (Bernie's) medical records without his consent.

- Explain consent issues as they apply to this case if required.

- Show empathy to Leonie's personal circumstances and her worries about the future.

- Explain that there could be various reasons for Bernie's apparent memory loss and that some screening tests are needed before an Alzheimer's diagnosis can be confirmed.

CHAPTER 5

KEY POINTS AND FURTHER READING

Dementia is an irreversible global impairment of cognitive function in the absence of reduced consciousness. One in five people aged >80 years is affected to some degree. There are various causes, with Alzheimer's disease being the most common. Vascular dementia generally causes a stepwise progression because significant vascular events occur; Lewy body dementia is characterised by parkinsonism and frontotemporal dementia affects personality without necessarily causing memory loss. Medication side effects and low mood causing pseudodementia are important causes to rule out. Standard screening tests aim to exclude treatable causes of confusion.

NICE. *Supporting People with Dementia and Their Carers in Health and Social Care.* London: NICE, 2006. www.nice.org.uk/guidance/CG42

This guideline summarises an approach to diagnosis, treatment, and support for dementia patients and their carers. The diagnosis should be confirmed by a specialist following an assessment comprising an appropriate cognitive test such as the Mini-Mental State Examination (MMSE) or the 6 Item Cognitive Impairment Test (6-CIT), blood tests and brain imaging. In practice, brain imaging is currently reserved for equivocal, early onset or non-Alzheimer-type dementias. Health and social care professionals should seek consent from people with dementia. This should entail informing the person of options, and checking that he or she understands that there is no coercion and he or she continues to consent over time. If the person lacks the capacity to make a decision, the provisions of the Mental Capacity Act 2005 come into play.

Anticholinesterase medications should be considered for mild–moderate dementia and started by a specialist, monitored 3 monthly in the first instance, and reviewed at least 6 monthly. They should be stopped once dementia becomes severe (MMSE 10 or less). Severe dementia patients might be offered memantine.

In elderly patients with dementia, antipsychotics increase the stroke risk. NICE guidance on dementia recommends that antipsychotics should be used only in exceptional circumstances, ie if severely distressed or in immediate risk of harm to themselves or others.

CHAPTER 5

Health and social care workers should assess the needs of carers as set out in the Carers and Disabled Children Act 2000 and the Carers (Equal Opportunities) Act 2004. These acts support the provision of psychological therapy including cognitive–behavioural therapy for carers who experience distress.

People with dementia may develop challenging behaviour as part of the progressive illness or for non-cognitive reasons such as occult infection, unidentified pain and medication side effects. Such changes should trigger prompt assessment. As time passes individually tailored care plans should assist carers in knowing how and when to call for help.

Mental Capacity Act 2005

www.publicguardian.gov.uk, click on 'Mental Capacity Act'

This Act of Parliament came into effect in 2007 and was created to protect the autonomy of the individual. It provides a legal framework for decision-making on behalf of adults, aged 16 years and older, who lack the capacity to make decisions themselves. It also provides guidance on how adults aged 18 years and older, who have capacity, can make 'advanced decisions' and how they might nominate a 'lasting power of attorney' (LPA) to make future health decisions on their behalf. When an individual who lacks capacity for a decision has no family, friends or nominated LPA, there is a duty to appoint an independent mental capacity advocate (IMCA) to help decide what constitutes 'best interests'. If and when there is conflict or concern about a decision the Court of Protection can be called upon to arbitrate.

Capacity is defined as a time- and decision-specific ability. This means that for each decision there should be a reassessment of capacity to perform the following:

- Able to understand information
- Able to retain information related to the decision to be made
- Able to use or weigh information as part of the decision-making process
- Able to communicate a decision by any means, including blinking or squeezing a hand.

CHAPTER 5

There are five core principles as follows:

1. A person must be assumed to have capacity until it is established that he or she lacks capacity.

2. A person is not to be treated as unable to make a decision unless all practicable (doable) steps to help him or her to do so have been taken without success.

3. A person is not to be treated as unable to make a decision merely because he or she makes an 'unwise' decision.

4. A decision made on behalf of a person who lacks capacity must be made in his or her best interests.

5. A decision made on behalf of a person who lacks capacity must be made in a way that is least restrictive of the person's rights and freedom of action.

Lack of capacity can be due to a range of causes, including unconsciousness, dementia, learning disabilities, stroke, head injuries or mental health problems.

CASE 7

INSTRUCTIONS TO THE CANDIDATE (CASE NOTES)

Name	Tomas Skolski
Age	53 years
Address	15 Grove Street, SL9 10PL
Social and family history	Lives with wife and two children
Past medical history	Osteoarthritis
Drug history	Nil
Current medication	Nil
Additional info (results/letters)	Nil

BRAINSTORM

INSTRUCTIONS TO THE ROLE PLAYER (PATIENT)

NOT TO BE SEEN BY THE CANDIDATE

Patient background:

You are 53-year-old Tomas Skolski and have come to the doctor because you cannot sleep, although in truth you are moderately depressed. You are neither suicidal nor psychotic. Your low mood has led you to drink heavily, but you are not physically addicted to alcohol. You would accept any help with your mood and your drinking.

You came to the UK from Poland 2 years ago with your wife and two school-age children, to try to make a better life. In Poland you had gained an IT PhD but there were no jobs. You have not found IT work here either, and have worked in supermarkets since your arrival.

You speak and act in a depressed manner.

Opening statement:

'Could I have some sleeping pills? I haven't slept properly for ages and it is really getting me down.'

Freely divulged in response to open questions:

Not sleeping is really getting you down.

Your wife complains that you are a miserable soul since you arrived in the UK.

You are probably drinking too much, but this is only to try to help you get to sleep, and to take your mind off not getting a decent job here in the UK.

Information divulged if asked specifically:

IT PhD in Poland, high-flyer.

Came to UK for better life and to find IT work.

Not sure why feeling down but probably because no IT work.

You display moderate depressive biological and psychological symptoms.

You are not suicidal, have no ideation of intent.

You do not have psychotic symptoms.

You get embarrassed that you work in a supermarket.

You feel guilty that you have not provided a better life for family.

You drink a quarter bottle of vodka per night (250 ml of 40% strength alcohol), and have done this for the last 2 years.

You would like to cut down but get angry if your wife suggests this, you feel guilty about the amount you drink, but do not have an eye opener, and regularly go several days without alcohol when working night shifts without symptoms of alcohol withdrawal (CAGE questions).

No other drug misuse.

NOTES

OVERALL AIM OF THE CASE

Identify the 'depressed' hidden agenda and deal with this as per UK guidelines.

Recognise alcohol as part of the problem and offer support for this.

Exploring the psychosocial landscape of this case is key to the optimal consultation.

Providing empathy and support is of paramount importance.

DATA GATHERING, TECHNICAL AND ASSESSMENT SKILLS

- Why does he think he is not sleeping, and what has he tried so far?

- Assess depression severity including risk to self and others. Use validated questionnaires, eg. PHQ-9/HAD

- Coexistent psychotic symptoms

- Assess alcohol history, ie units/week, AUDIT questionnaire, symptoms of withdrawal.

- Assess using CAGE questions: Have you felt you should **c**ut down you drinking? Do you feel **a**ngry/annoyed when people comment on your drinking? Have you felt **g**uilty about your drinking habits? Have you ever had a drink in the morning (**e**ye-opener)?

- Does he want help giving up/cutting down alcohol?

- Biopsychosocial background

- Other drug use

- Past history of mental problems

- Other medical conditions that might exacerbate low mood.

CLINICAL MANAGEMENT SKILLS

- Sleep hygiene suggestions framed in the context of depressed alcohol misuser

- Depression management as per NICE guidelines, ie lifestyle measures, self-help, psychological intervention, medication options

- Consider a fit note for time off work

- Options for treatment and support of excessive drinking

- Plans for follow-up and safety-netting, ie usually see again within a 2-week time frame.

INTERPERSONAL SKILLS

- Active listening skills to demonstrate your attention and concern, eg nod your head, lean towards the patient, echo his words, mirror his body language, summarise to show that you have listened and to check your understanding of his situation.

- Use silences to give the patient time to express his emotions.

- Respond to verbal and physical clues, eg if a patient 'looks down' then comment that he 'looks down', OR if he uses a phrase that refers to his mental state, repeat it back to him to acknowledge that you heard him expressing this.

- Explain your diagnosis of depression and excessive alcohol use.

- Display empathy while maintaining professional objectivity.

- Ask questions in a sensitive manner, eg 'How bad have you felt ... have you got so low that you have thought of harming yourself ... or made any plans to do this?'

KEY POINTS AND FURTHER READING

NICE. *Depression – The treatment and management of depression in adults.* London: NICE, 2009. www.nice.org.uk/guidance/CG90

Depression is a heterogeneous diagnosis, characterised by low mood and/ or loss of pleasure in most activities. It is recommended that we screen for depression opportunistically and in high-risk groups by asking if a person has felt down and/or found little pleasure in doing things in the last month. If the answer to either of these questions is in the affirmative, a fuller depression assessment should be made.

Severity of depression should be determined using the criteria of the *Diagnostic and Statistical Manual of Mental Disorders* (DSM-IV) which take account of the number and severity of symptoms and also the degree of functional impairment. In brief, the DSM-IV criteria define depression as follows:

- Presence of at least one of the following three states which interferes with the person's life: abnormal depressed mood most of the day, nearly every day, for at least 2 weeks OR abnormal loss of all interest and pleasure most of the day, nearly every day, for at least 2 weeks OR, if 18 or younger, abnormal irritable mood most of the day, nearly every day, for at least 2 weeks.

- At least five of the following symptoms have been present during the same 2-week depressed period:
  - abnormal depressed mood OR irritable mood if a child or adolescent
  - abnormal loss of interest and pleasure
  - appetite or weight disturbance
  - sleep disturbance
  - activity disturbance, either abnormal agitation or abnormal slowing
  - abnormal loss of energy
  - abnormal self-reproach or inappropriate guilt
  - abnormal poor concentration or indecisiveness

CHAPTER 5

- abnormal morbid thoughts of death (not just fear of dying) or suicide.

The DSM-IV criteria classify depression as follows:

- Subthreshold depressive symptoms = fewer than five symptoms

- Mild depression = few, if any, symptoms in excess of the five required to make the diagnosis, and symptoms result in only minor functional impairment

- Moderate depression = symptoms or functional impairment is between 'mild' and 'severe'

- Severe depression = most symptoms, and the symptoms markedly interfere with functioning. Can occur with or without psychotic symptoms.

NICE outline specific management paths for the different severities of depression:

- Subthreshold and mild depression: low-intensity psychosocial interventions, guided by the patient's preference:

  - a structured group physical activity programme

  - a group-based peer support (self-help) programme

  - individual guided self-help based on the principles of cognitive–behavioural therapy (CBT)

  - computerised CBT.

- Persisting subthreshold or mild depression for at least 2 years and moderate and severe depression:

  - psychosocial interventions as for mild depression

  - group-based CBT

  - individual CBT

  - behavioural couples therapy for people who have a regular partner and where the relationship may contribute to the development or maintenance of depression, or where involving the partner is considered to be of potential therapeutic benefit

  - antidepressant drugs.

CHAPTER 5

As part of the Quality and Outcomes Framework (QOF 2013–14), it is also important to record a biopsychosocial history on the day that you diagnose depression. This covers the above and includes quality of personal relationships, social support, living conditions, employment or financial worries, current or previous substance or alcohol use, previous treatments and response to treatment.

NICE. *Alcohol-use disorders: Diagnosis, assessment and management of harmful drinking and alcohol dependence.* London: NICE, 2011. www.nice. org.uk/guidance/CG115

These guidelines classify and define alcohol disorders as:

• Hazardous drinking: pattern of alcohol use that increases a person's risk of social, psychological or physical harm

• Harmful drinking: pattern of drinking that results in harm

• Alcohol dependence: behavioural, cognitive and physical signs that indicate a difficulty in controlling consumption such that alcohol is given a higher priority than other activities and obligations.

It is judged that about one in four adults has an alcohol disorder as defined by this guidance.

Screening using validated questionnaires is recommended for people with an increased risk of harm. Validated questionnaires include AUDIT (alcohol use disorders identification tool) and not the CAGE questions. There are 10 AUDIT questions. If someone answers the first three screening questions (AUDIT-C or shortened version) such that they typically drink a maximum of one to two alcoholic drinks at a single sitting, and drink six or more alcoholic drinks at a single sitting a maximum of once a month, they are deemed low risk and need not answer the subsequent seven questions.

Interventions are tailored to the severity of the problem and the individual's circumstances, and are expected to be provided by appropriately-trained professionals:

• Harmful and mild alcohol dependence: psychological intervention such as CBT.

CHAPTER 5

- Severe alcohol dependence: offer additional assisted alcohol withdrawal which should be residential under specified high risk circumstances. Also, offer interventions to promote abstinence after successful withdrawal, including medications such as acamprosate and ongoing psychological therapies.

- Misuse of alcohol aged 10–17 years: consider offering CBT and / or family therapy.

Previous related guidelines also discuss specific physical complications of alcohol-use disorders:

- Acute alcohol withdrawal: admit those in acute withdrawal and consider lorazepam as first line for treating delirium tremens, provide support and refer those at high risk of withdrawal to specialist services where detoxification regimen using chlordiazepoxide or diazepam can be prescribed and overseen.

- Wernicke's encephalopathy: prevent by offering thiamine (and other B-vitamin supplements) to those in specified high-risk groups.

- Alcohol-related liver disease: exclude other causes of liver dysfunction, refer to a liver specialist to consider biopsy if dysfunction seemingly irreversible; consider referral for transplantation if there is persistent liver dysfunction after best management and abstinence from alcohol for at least 3 months.

- Alcohol-related pancreatitis: check pancreatic exocrine and endocrine function, use CT as first-line imaging modality, refer if in pain or if considering pancreatic enzyme supplementation.

CHAPTER 5

CASE 8

INSTRUCTIONS TO THE CANDIDATE (CASE NOTES)

Name	Bryony Leighton
Age	15 years
Address	Hillside House, Borrowcop Lane, High Wycombe
Social and family history	Lives with parents and sister Hannah
Past medical history	Asthma
Current medication	Nil
Additional info (results/letters)	Nil

BRAINSTORM

EXAMINATION FINDINGS

Information offered on iPad if appropriate. The examiner will pass this information to the candidate when he or she offers to examine BP, weight and height.

- BMI 24

- BP 128/74

INSTRUCTIONS TO THE ROLE PLAYER (PATIENT)

NOT TO BE SEEN BY THE CANDIDATE

Patient background:

You are 15-year-old Bryony Leighton, an intelligent 15 year old who is confidentially attending to request the combined oral contraceptive pill (COC). You have been with your 16-year-old boyfriend from school for over a year, and have recently started having sex together. Up until now you have used condoms, have not had any problems, but think that a COC would be a surer way of preventing pregnancy. Your older sister takes Microgynon 30 and this would be your first choice. You have not considered long-acting reversible contraceptives (LARCs) or alternatives, but they would not appeal to you. You do not want your parents to know, especially your father who is the local vicar.

THE CANDIDATE WILL NOT EXAMINE YOU BUT WILL BE HANDED A PIECE OF PAPER WITH THE 'FINDINGS' IF HE OR SHE OFFERS AN EXAMINATION

Opening statement:

'My sister told me I should talk to you. I would like to go on the pill.'

Freely divulged in response to open questions:

1-year relationship with 16-year-old boyfriend from school.

Started having sex together using condoms about a month ago.

Neither of your parents knows that you have started having sex, and your parents do not know that you are seeing the doctor today.

Information divulged if asked specifically:

Menarche aged 13 years.

Regular periods, K 5/28.

Day 21 of current period.

Only ever had sex with boyfriend and think that he has only ever had sex with you.

No pregnancies.

No STI (sexually transmitted infection) symptoms or past history.

No contraindications to COC.

Have not considered alternatives, including LARCs, though none appeals if offered.

NOTES

OVERALL AIM OF THE CASE

Recognise the ethical dimension of this case with its focus on the assessment of Gillick competence.

There is a lot of information to cover if a complete assessment is to be made, as well as starting a COC, so realistic time management can often be an issue with this apparently 'simple' scenario.

Consider contraindications to use of COC.

Provide the information required to achieve a safe 'pill start'.

DATA GATHERING, TECHNICAL AND ASSESSMENT SKILLS

- Social history

- Menstrual history

- Sexual history

- Details of current relationship

- Could she be pregnant already?

- Was she hoping to start the pill today?

- Exclude contraindications to COC use

- Has she considered LARCs/alternatives?

- BP and BMI.

CHAPTER 5

CLINICAL MANAGEMENT SKILLS

- Assess Gillick competence according to the Fraser guidelines
- Encourage involvement of parents
- Offer LARCs as options
- Start discussion on the pill: pros/cons of COC use (ensuring that you mention cancer and clotting risks as potential downsides, but making sure that you also mention positive attributes such as overall cancer risk reduction, and regular, usually lighter menses), when to start, 7-day rule, extra protection with condoms/abstinence, illness, medication changes, how to take, missed pill, STI, GP review.

INTERPERSONAL SKILLS

- Appreciate that this is a potentially embarrassing scenario for a young woman
- Non-patronising
- Reassure the patient of the confidential nature of your discussion
- Why is she attending now? Is she worried that she might already be pregnant?
- Can she be encouraged to involve her parents and, if not, why not?

KEY POINTS AND FURTHER READING

About one in four people in the UK will have sex before the age of 16 years.

GMC. *0–18 years: Guidance for all doctors*. 2007. www.gmc-uk.org/guidance/

This guidance is informed by several Acts of Parliament and by consensus professional opinion:

- The Children's Act 1989 (amended 2004) defines the child as a person under the age of 18 years. Its central tenet is to act in the 'best interests' of the child.

- The Sexual Offences Act 2003 which came into force in 2004 says that mutually consensual sexual relations can be legal for individuals from 13 years to 16 years, so long as there is no abuse or exploitation, and as long as participants are of a similar age. From 16 years to 18 years, individuals are still protected under this law and consideration still needs to be given to possible exploitation through prostitution or abuse of power. Thus there is an obligation to discuss all cases aged under 13 years with colleagues and consider whether involvement of child protection authorities is in the child's best interests. These discussions must be documented. Practices and professionals working with children must be aware of their local child protection referral pathways.

Fraser Guidelines: *Gillick vs West Norfolk and Wisbech Area Health Authority* 1985

In 1985, Lord Fraser issued guidance to doctors and other health professionals about when contraceptive advice/treatment can be given to a person under 16 without parental consent. The 'Fraser Guidelines' have become a byword for assessment of capacity to consent in patients under 16. 'Gillick competence' has similarly become a byword for this situation as it pertains to provision of contraception. Before providing contraception advice/treatment a health professional must be satisfied that:

- the young person understands the advice
- the young person cannot be persuaded to tell his or her parents or allow the doctor to tell them that she is seeking contraceptive advice
- the young person is likely to begin or continue having unprotected sex with or without contraceptive treatment
- the young person's physical or mental health is likely to suffer unless he or she receives contraceptive advice or treatment.

UKMEC (UK Medical eligibility criteria) – for the COC. www.fpa.org.uk

CHAPTER 5

CASE 9: HOME VISIT

INSTRUCTIONS TO THE CANDIDATE (CASE NOTES)

Name	Arthur Carlton
Age	82 years
Address	20 Ringmore Rise, High Wycombe
Social and family history	Lives with wife, ex-smoker (1980, 20/day)
Past medical history	Hypertension
	Type 2 diabetes
	Myocardial infarction
	Left total hip replacement
Current medication	Atenolol
	Simvastatin
	Ramipril
	Metformin
	Co-codamol 30/500
Additional info (results/letters)	Consultation notes for a surgery appointment 2 days ago:

'4d cough, non-productive, no cp/fever/leg symptoms

O/E sats 95%, RR 18, HR 80 reg, pink throat, chest clear all zones.

Impression: viral URTI

Plan: conservative measures, review if worse, not better within a week, or any other concerns

BRAINSTORM

EXAMINATION FINDINGS

Information offered on iPad if appropriate. The examiner will pass these findings to the candidate following their examination, if it is done.

- Oriented
- 38.2°C
- Capillary refill time (CRT) 2 s
- Well hydrated
- BP 92/54 mmHg
- HR 96 reg
- RR 38
- Sats 90% in air
- Marked intercostal recession, dyspnoeic at rest
- Dull percussion note and bronchial breathing left base
- Heart sounds normal
- Legs + arms no signs of DVT.

INSTRUCTIONS TO THE ROLE PLAYER (PATIENT)

NOT TO BE SEEN BY THE CANDIDATE

Patient background:

You are 82-year-old Arthur Carlton. You have had a cough for almost a week, and are feeling increasingly feverish and short of breath, even at rest. You saw your own GP in the surgery 2 days ago and were told that you had a viral illness but to call if things got worse or persisted for longer than a week.

Two days later, you are too weak to leave your home, can barely make the trip to the toilet and are worried by the sharp pain on the left side of your chest each time that you breathe in deeply. You had an MI many years ago and, although the pain is different, you worry that you have had another MI.

You are half expecting the doctor to send you to hospital to treat an MI. You detest feeling weak, and appearances are important to you. As such, you try to make light of how unwell you are, and feel uncomfortable with the doctor seeing you in your bed clothes.

The doctor will be expected to offer to examine you. This will include examination of the chest for which exposure of the skin is expected.

AT THE END OF THEIR EXAMINATION THE CANDIDATE WILL BE HANDED A PIECE OF PAPER WITH THE EXAMINATION FINDINGS THAT WILL 'CONFIRM' A LIKELY CHEST INFECTION.

Opening statement:

(BREATHLESS) 'It's so good of you to come doctor. I really don't feel at all good.'

Freely divulged in response to open questions:

Cough started a week ago.

Saw Dr Redican a couple of days ago, and were told that you probably had a virus.

Sorry to have to ask for a home visit but told to do so if felt worse.

Feeling increasingly weak, hot and cold, coughing up green phlegm, and now got a sharp pain in the chest every time that you inhale.

Had an MI about 20 years ago, and just wonder if it's the same again.

Information divulged if asked specifically:

Describe the chest pain as sharp, no haemoptysis/DVT symptoms.

Barely able to get out of bed due to shortness of breath and pain on inspiration.

Not sleeping.

You live with your wife who is 'downstairs'.

Your wife will be fine alone in the home if you need to be admitted.

Regular meds = atenolol, simvastatin, ramipril, metformin, co-codamol 30/500.

Medical history = hypertension, type 2 diabetes, MI 1980 (gave up smoking), left THR.

You think that it is another MI and half expect to be sent to hospital for this.

NOTES

OVERALL AIM OF THE CASE

Show a professional approach to the consultation in a home environment, and to recognise the clinical indication for hospital admission.

There is a focus in this case on targeted data gathering, appropriate management of a 'high-risk' pneumonia, and the interpersonal skills to explain the examination that you wish to perform, the diagnosis and the recommended management to an elderly patient who had expected to be admitted but for different reasons.

DATA GATHERING, TECHNICAL AND ASSESSMENT SKILLS

- Clarify duration of illness
- Characterise chest pain: pleuritic, no DVT/pulmonary embolism (PE) symptoms, not cardiac
- Past medical history
- Is the patient a smoker?
- Impact on daily activities and sleep
- ICE.

CLINICAL MANAGEMENT SKILLS

CRB65 would suggest that this patient has a significant mortality risk and so should be admitted for intravenous antibiotics in secondary care.

CHAPTER 5

INTERPERSONAL SKILLS

- Act politely in another person's home.

- You are consulting a person in bed, maybe in his pyjamas; act with due deference to his personal boundaries and show respect for any discomfort that he may feel in this situation.

- Ask the patient's permission to 'measure his blood pressure, listen to his lungs and check his breathing'.

- Explain the diagnosis and the recommended management in patient-friendly language

KEY POINTS AND FURTHER READING

British Thoracic Society. *Guidelines for the Management of Community Acquired Pneumonia in Adults*. 2009. *Thorax*, Vol 64, Supplement III, www.brit-thoracic.org.uk

There are take-home messages for community-based health professionals:

- Clinical judgement, and the CRB65 score, should be used to decide whether to treat patients at home or in hospital.

- Review patients treated in the community after 48 hours, or earlier if indicated.

- Patients should be advised to rest, drink plenty of fluids and not to smoke.

- Use simple analgesia such as paracetamol for pleuritic pain.

- Pulse oximetry should be used and be available in the out-of-hours setting.

- Amoxicillin 500 mg tds is the preferred antibiotic, with doxycycline or clarithromycin as second-line alternative.

- Microbiological investigations are not recommended routinely but may be appropriate in patients who do not respond to empirical antibiotic therapy.

- Patients with suspected, severe, life-threatening community-acquired pneumonia referred to hospital should be given antibiotics in the community: either benzylpenicillin 1.2 g intravenously or amoxicillin 1 g orally.

The CRB65 score used in the BTS guidelines comes from a cohort study by Lim et al, published in *Thorax* in 2003: www.ncbi.nlm.nih.gov/pubmed/12728155

One point is awarded for each of the following features:

- **C**onfusion – Mental Test Score (MTS) <8/10, or new disorientation in person, place, time

- **R**espiratory rate $\geq$ 30 breaths/min

- **B**lood pressure – systolic of $\leq$90 mmHg or a diastolic of $\leq$60 mmHg

- **A**ge $\geq$**65** years.

It found that the risk of death for people with:

- a score of 0 was 1.2%

- a score of 1 was 5.3%

- a score of 2 was 12.2%

- a score of 3 was 18.2%

- a score of 4 was 32.9%.

The recommended management for individuals according to their CRB-65 score is:

- **CRB-65 score of $\geq$3**: urgent admission to hospital

- **CRB-65 score of 1–2**: consider same-day assessment in secondary care

- **CRB-65 score of 0:** treatment at home is usually appropriate, depending on *clinical judgement* and available social support

- A systematic review and meta-analysis showed (McNally P Ervine E Shields MD et al. *Br J Gen Pract* 2010;60:770) that, in the primary care setting, the tool overestimated risk, leading to inappropriate admissions

- The SIGN and BTS guideline on the management of asthma recommend that anyone with asthma and oxygen saturation of < 92% should be admitted to hospital (SIGN and BTS, 2009).

CHAPTER 5

CASE 10

INSTRUCTIONS TO THE CANDIDATE (CASE NOTES)

Name	William Baxendale
Age	56 years
Address	5 Ruston Cottage, High Wycombe
Social and family history	Lives with wife
Past medical history	OA
	Essential hypertension
Current medication	Bendroflumethiazide
	Lisinopril
	Simvastatin
	Paracetamol
	Naproxen
	Omeprazole
Additional info (results/letters)	
Most recent results (fasting)	Hb 13.4
	WBC 9.2
	Platelets 290
	Na$^+$ 139
	K$^+$ 4.5
	Creatinine 120
	eGFR 68
	Total cholesterol 3.9
	HDL 3.0
	LDL 1.9

TG 2.1

Fasting blood glucose 5.3

LFTs – normal ranges

Urine ACR 0.7

BRAINSTORM

EXAMINATION FINDINGS

Information offered on iPad if appropriate. These findings are given to the candidate if he or she offers to examine the patient. An examination will not be performed.

BP 138/78.

Multiple pigmented moles over back – benign appearances, no regional lymph node enlargement.

INSTRUCTIONS TO THE ROLE PLAYER (PATIENT)

NOT TO BE SEEN BY THE CANDIDATE

Patient background:

You are 56-year-old William Baxendale. You have not been to the GP for 6 months and have 'helpfully' saved up all of your problems for a single visit. You would like to deal with each of these complaints, but are particularly worried about the moles on your back as you have a friend who recently had a skin cancer removed.

The other complaints are of less concern.

You will happily prioritise your list of requests if the GP deals with you in a patient-centred manner.

The candidate is being tested on time management among other things, and you are a 'rambling' type of patient who will 'frustrate' the doctor by adding detail to each question answered, thereby making his or her job harder with respect to keeping to time.

THE CANDIDATE WILL NOT EXAMINE YOU AND HE OR SHE WILL BE HANDED A PIECE OF PAPER WITH 'EXAMINATION FINDINGS' ON IF HE OR SHE OFFERS TO EXAMINE YOUR MOLES OR TO MEASURE YOUR BLOOD PRESSURE.

Opening statement:

'I haven't been here for ages so there a few things I'd like to get sorted please.'

Freely divulged in response to open questions:

(IN A RAMBLING STYLE)

Need some more medicines because you have run out.

Would like your blood pressure checked.

Would like to hear through the results of the blood and urine tests that you had a few months ago.

Your left shoulder is no better after a steroid injection last year.

Might have a bit of a cold coming on because sneezing a lot in last 2 days.

Please check moles on back.

Information divulged if asked specifically:

If asked to list 'all the things you wanted to deal with today', succinctly list them without embellishment.

If asked to prioritise your list, again, succinctly list them without embellishment with moles as your primary concern.

With respect to moles: no changes, attends now because wife prompted and worried because a friend had 'skin cancer' excised recently, no past history of skin cancer, no high-risk childhood UV exposure, lived in UK all life, never worked outdoors, no family history skin/related cancers.

With respect to shoulder: onset 1 year ago, unclear precipitant, no limitation in activities, steroid injection 6 months ago worked for about 3 months, generally better, but keen to have another steroid injection or discuss options.

Live with wife.

NOTES

OVERALL AIM OF THE CASE

The challenge is to manage the 10 minutes allowed in an optimal manner.

Time manage the consultation but allow the patient to prioritise his complaints to achieve a patient-centred consultation.

DATA GATHERING, TECHNICAL AND ASSESSMENT SKILLS

- Identify the patient's priorities
- Identify 'all' the patient's concerns to avoid missing something urgent
- Take an appropriate clinical history excluding red flags with respect to 'moles'.

CLINICAL MANAGEMENT SKILLS

- Prioritising the list of concerns with the patient allows you to identify any potentially urgent problems as well as the patient's agenda.
- Management of benign pigmented moles: explain and safety net.
- Management of hypertension with the information provided, ie no immediate action needed, advise regular BP monitoring.
- Shared management plan, including plans for possible future consultations.
- Explain that often easier and safer to deal with one or two problems at a time, or that he might consider making a double appointment if he has more than one problem to cover in a consultation.

CHAPTER 5

INTERPERSONAL SKILLS

- Patient-centred approach by allowing the patient to prioritise his concerns.

- Explain that he can have multiple consultations if required.

- Why attending now?

- Does he think that he might have a skin cancer like his friend?

- What was he expecting to achieve from the consultation?

- What are his social circumstances?

- People with 'multiple problems' tend to present in this way for several common reasons: among others these include those who have busy working lives with little time to get to see their doctor, stress and low mood, and rare attenders who do not understand how the 10-minute consultation system is set up.

KEY POINTS AND FURTHER READING

Time is among the most precious resources that we have in dealing with our patients. We should aim to make efficient use of this finite resource and advise further consultations when appropriate. There are diverse strategies for making effective use of time in the consultation and these are comprehensively covered by the body of literature on the 'consultation model'.

A few basic time management strategies include:

- Determine the patient's agenda and his reason for attendance at the outset.

- A period of open questioning at the start of the consultation facilitates the expression of the patient's ideas, concerns and expectations.

- Use direct questioning with respect to ideas, concerns and expectations if they are not volunteered spontaneously.

CHAPTER 5

- Summarise your understanding of the patient's attendance to ensure a 'shared' understanding and that there are no patient concerns that you may have missed.

- Future appointment if the patient's concerns are not covered at a single sitting.

- Be realistic with the time available.

Useful phrases that may assist in achieving these goals are as follows:

- What has brought you in today?

- What were you hoping to get out of today's visit?

- Is there anything else that you wanted to cover today?

- What would your priorities be?

- Is there anything that could wait for another day?

- To deal with these concerns properly, could we give ourselves a bit more time by arranging to see each other again?

Tate P. *The Doctor's Communication Handbook*. Radcliffe, 2006.

Pendleton et al. *The New Consultation: Developing doctor-patient communication*. OUP, 2003.

www.skillscascade.com/models.htm

Useful website summarising and referencing landmark works on the consultation.

CASE 11

INSTRUCTIONS TO THE CANDIDATE (CASE NOTES)

Name   Jessica Isaacs

Age   23 years

Address   17 Allington Avenue, Bourne End, SL9 1DL

Social and family history   Father died from AAA rupture

Mother died last month from MI

Past medical history   Nil

Drug history   Microgynon 30

Additional info (results/letters)   Last consultation (nurse):

'Palpitations. No chest pains. For last 4 weeks. For Hb, U&Es, TFTs and ECG. See GP for f/u'

Results   ECG report from cardiology email reporting service:

'Sinus rhythm with single ventricular ectopic. Refer to cardiology if red flag symptoms.'

CHAPTER 5

BRAINSTORM

EXAMINATION FINDINGS

Information offered on iPad if appropriate, ie if candidate offers to examine the heart and take the blood pressure.

BP 112/76

Regular pulse 72 bpm

HS normal, nil added

RR 12/min

Chest bases clear

JVP normal waveform

Sats 98%

INSTRUCTIONS TO THE ROLE PLAYER (PATIENT)

NOT TO BE SEEN BY THE CANDIDATE

Patient background:

You are a 23-year-old medical student, Jessica Isaacs. You have experienced a fluttering sensation in the chest for the last 5 weeks. You are petrified that you are going to have a heart attack because your mother died recently of an MI at the age of 62, and your father died a few years ago aged 65 from a ruptured abdominal aortic aneurysm. You're still grieving the loss of both your parents. You have just started your medical studies as a mature student, and essentially have no medical knowledge yet.

(The candidate will be handed a piece of paper with examination findings if he or she offers to examine you. An examination will not be done.)

Opening statement:

(WORRIED DEMEANOUR)

'I've come for my heart test results, but I'm still getting these chest flutters.'

Freely divulged in response to open questions:

You have been experiencing palpitations for the last 5 weeks.

The nurse organised some tests and you've come to get the results.

You're very anxious and are convinced that you'll have a heart attack.

You're mum died recently from a heart attack, a 'myocardial in-something'.

Information divulged if asked specifically:

Intermittent 'fluttering' in your chest, usually at night.

They never occur when you exercise.

The palpitations never last more than a few seconds.

No associated chest pain, breathlessness, dizziness or fainting.

You don't have diarrhoea.

You don't sweat or wheeze.

Your weight is stable.

You don't take illicit drugs.

You drink a lot of caffeine; you've had to stay up late to study.

You take the pill.

You have heard of atrial ectopics but can't remember what they mean. You're only in pre-clinical school having done an economics degree first.

You accept that you are anxious, but do not feel a need for help.

You don't suffer from any other anxiety symptoms.

You feel very low about your mum's death, but are not surprised that she died at a relatively young age because she smoked and was overweight.

You aren't suicidal.

You would be happy to have a 24-hour monitor if offered.

CHAPTER 5

NOTES

OVERALL AIM OF THE CASE

Deal with a common presentation, excluding the red flags required to make a safe assessment of a benign cardiac condition, while handling the patient's anxiety.

DATA GATHERING, TECHNICAL AND ASSESSMENT SKILLS

- What does she mean by 'chest flutters'?

- Cardiac history and characterisation of the palpitations covering red flag symptoms such as association with exercise, syncope, chest pain, shortness of breath, and family history of sudden death

- Drug history

- Recreational drugs, alcohol and caffeine

- Symptoms of thyroid disease

- Risk factors for cardiovascular disease

- Clinical examination of cardiovascular status.

CLINICAL MANAGEMENT SKILLS

- Confess to the need for further assistance if you are unsure about how to manage a presentation: this might involve asking a colleague and getting back to the patient, or could justify referral to secondary care for a second opinion

- Offer support and options for managing the patient's anxiety

- Suggest cutting down on stimulants, eg coffee

- Ectopics, both atrial and ventricular, are usually benign and rarely need treating

- Have you addressed her needs?

- Follow-up?

CHAPTER 5

INTERPERSONAL SKILLS

- Explain in patient-friendly language, educating and checking understanding.

- Empathise by acknowledging verbal and non-verbal cues, eg 'You sound anxious'. Attempt to understand the sources and her degree of anxiety.

- Does she imagine that she will have the same problem as either/both parents?

- Don't assume knowledge, ie this medical student may not have medical knowledge.

- Offer a chaperone if examining a female patient involving exposure of the chest wall.

- What was she expecting, ie referral to a specialist?

KEY POINTS AND FURTHER READING

Thakkar R. *The basics – palpitations*, 2009. www.GPonline.com, 2009.

www.cks.nhs.uk, search 'palpitations' in 'Clinical Topics'

Management of patients with palpitations at the time of consulting in primary care:

- Known heart problem that could predispose to a dangerous arrhythmia?

- Red flag symptoms suggesting a serious complication?

  - breathlessness?

  - chest pain?

  - syncope/presyncope?

- Check blood pressure, pulse rhythm, rate and character

CHAPTER 5

- 12-lead ECG, including a long rhythm strip which may demonstrate:
  - ventricular tachycardia (VT)
  - supraventricular tachycardia (SVT)
  - sinus tachycardia
  - bradycardia
  - atrial fibrillation
  - atrial flutter
  - extrasystoles (atrial and ventricular)
  - congenital structural disorders

Admit as an emergency and send with ECG if:

- Cardiac-type pain ± failure with palpitations
- Unable to exclude VT or SVT

Consider cardiology referral for stable patients without palpitations at the time of consulting:

- Symptoms suggestive of VT or SVT
- Red flag symptoms with palpitations = cardiac-type chest pain, shortness of breath, syncope and presyncope, exercise-induced, family history of sudden cardiac death
- Evidence of major structural heart disease
- Captured abnormality on a 12-lead ECG.

Patients who may not require referral:

- Patients with symptoms of extrasystoles (missed beats followed by a strong beat, most noticeable at rest) if there is no evidence of ischaemic heart disease, major structural heart disease or major ECG abnormalities.
- Patients with sinus tachycardia may not need referral provided that systematic examination is undertaken and appropriate investigations are arranged to exclude underlying causes (eg anaemia, heart failure, medication, chronic lung disease, thyrotoxicosis).

CHAPTER 5

CASE 12

INSTRUCTIONS TO THE CANDIDATE (CASE NOTES)

Name	Barbara Parry
Age	24 years
Address	32 Gable Croft, London W5
Social and family history	Nil
Past medical history	Borderline personality disorder
Current medication	Nil
Additional info (results/letters)	Nil

BRAINSTORM

INSTRUCTIONS TO THE ROLE PLAYER (PATIENT)

NOT TO BE SEEN BY THE CANDIDATE

Patient background:

You are 24-year-old Barbara Parry. You work in a shoe shop. You are desperate to have a baby, and have been trying for 4 months. You have been with your 38-year-old partner Ben Leighton for 5 months, and he does not know that you have stopped taking the pill and are trying to get pregnant. You know that he had fertility investigations in a previous relationship and that he has never had children. You would like to know your partner's sperm sample results, are unaware of confidentiality disallowing this, and get upset and angry if the doctor refuses. If the doctor refuses to give you your partner's results, you ask for a referral to the fertility clinic, and are angry all over again if this is refused. You remain angry to the end if your requests are not met, you refuse to take no for an answer, and threaten to report the GP to the authorities unless you get the results.

Opening statement:

'I'm trying to get pregnant but it's just not happening for us. My partner has had a sperm test and I'd like to know the results please.'

Freely divulged in response to open questions:

You are concerned that you are nearly 25 and still not pregnant.

You have been in a relationship for 5 months and are desperate to have a baby.

You have been trying to get pregnant for 4 months.

Information divulged if asked specifically:

Your periods are regular 5/28 and your period started today.

You have had two uncomplicated first trimester terminations for social reasons.

Your partner Ben does not know that you have come for his sperm result today.

Ben does not know that you stopped taking the pill 4 months ago.

You are worried that your terminations may have caused you to be infertile but also suspect that the 'problem' may lie with Ben.

You do not smoke, drink moderately, are taking folic acid tablets and had a smear 6 months ago which was normal.

NOTES

OVERALL AIM OF THE CASE

Maintain confidentiality, and stick to your guns in the face of vociferous objection

Dealing with an angry patient

Attempt to educate the patient regarding fertility issues.

DATA GATHERING, TECHNICAL AND ASSESSMENT SKILLS

- Obstetric history including cause for terminations
- Menstrual history
- STI history
- Abdominal surgical history
- Drug history
- Social history including occupation, recreational drugs and alcohol use
- Family history of fertility problems
- Smear and rubella status
- Partner's fertility history
- How often are the couple having sex and is it vaginal sex with ejaculation?

CLINICAL MANAGEMENT SKILLS

- Maintain confidentiality
- Infertility tests are not indicated before a couple have been trying for at least 12 months under normal circumstances
- Preconception advice, ie folic acid, smoking, alcohol, drugs, exercise, weight, diet
- Advise intercourse two to three times/week.

CHAPTER 5

223

INTERPERSONAL SKILLS

- Be clear about confidentiality and the indications for fertility testing

- Avoid overt confrontation with an angry patient

- Are there other reasons why she has attended now?

- Check understanding of infertility and fertility rates according to age

- What are her worries?

- Attempt to reassure, ie about 90 per cent of healthy couples conceive within 12 months

- If she has regular periods then she is likely to be fertile

- Offer to meet the patient with her partner to discuss these issues, ideally after 1 year of trying together.

KEY POINTS AND FURTHER READING

GMC Confidentiality 2009. www.gmc-uk.org/guidance.

This guidance covers the following issues:

- Principles of confidentiality

- How to protect confidential information

- Disclosures without consent

- Public interest

- Patients who lack capacity to consent

- Sharing information with partners, carers, relatives and friends.

With reference to the scenario encountered in our case, a patient can expect that information about her in her medical records is held confidentially, unless she consents to sharing of information or if there is a qualified reason for a breach of that confidentiality. Such exceptions to disclosure without consent include circumstances required by law and when acting in the public interest.

CHAPTER 5

NICE. *Fertility: Assessment and treatment for people with fertility problems*, 2013. www.nice.org.uk/CG156

This guidance defines infertility as failure to conceive after regular unprotected sexual intercourse for 2 years in the absence of known reproductive pathology. A couple should be offered further clinical assessment and investigation.

Initial advice to people concerned about delays in conception:

- Cumulative likelihood of pregnancy is 80% after 1 year and 92% after 2 years
- Fertility declines with a woman's age such that a woman has a 94% chance of pregnancy if trying for 3 years at age 35 compared with 77% chance of the same at age 38 years
- Sexual intercourse every 2–3 days
- Not recommended to time sex with ovulation because this can increase stress
- Less than 2 units of alcohol twice a week for women and less than 4 units a day for men
- Avoid smoking, caffeine and recreational drugs
- Ideal BMI 19–29
- Offer a rubella screen and cervical smear if appropriate.

Early investigation and referral of infertility (before 12 months):

- women aged 36 or over
- HIV
- there is a known clinical cause of infertility or a history of predisposing factors for fertility.

Investigation and referral of infertility after 12 months of trying:

- Arrange blood tests to check ovulation and semen analysis
- Referral to specialist fertility centre

The guidance provides lots of information on how subsequent fertility investigations and treatment should be performed in secondary and tertiary centres. The age limit of referral has gone up to 42, provided that the woman meets certain criteria (there may be local variances to these guidelines).

CASE 13

INSTRUCTIONS TO THE CANDIDATE (CASE NOTES)

Name	Charangit Dheer
Age	59 years
Address	18 Gaia Lane, Bourne End, SL1 1PA
Family history	Diabetes
Social history	Lives with wife and two children
Past medical history	Nil
Drug history	Tamsulosin 400 mcg od
Additional info (results/letters)	Last consultation 2 weeks ago:

'Lower urinary tract symptoms, 1 year, getting worse, terminal dribbling, hesitancy, nocturia (3×/night). No features of diabetes. No dysuria. No back pain.

Abdo NAD. DRE large, smooth prostate, with no malignant features

Plan – MSU, glucose, PSA. Review GP 2 weeks, consider tamsulosin/finasteride.'

Results	MSU – no growth
	Glucose 6.0 mmol/l
	PSA 113 ng/ml (<4)

BRAINSTORM

INSTRUCTIONS TO THE ROLE PLAYER (PATIENT)

NOT TO BE SEEN BY THE CANDIDATE

Patient background:

You are 59-year-old Charangit Dheer, a solicitor. The doctor will be 'breaking bad news' that you have a high prostate blood test (prostate-specific antigen or PSA), which will mean little to you. It will also be unexpected.

You saw another doctor 2 weeks ago because of worsening lower urinary tract symptoms (LUTS) over the preceding 1 year. This doctor told you that you had a large 'prostate' which might be causing your urinary problems, although you needed a couple of tests to check your prostate and to check for diabetes before the best treatment could be advised.

You fully expect to be told that you have diabetes because your sister has just been diagnosed with this, and she had similar symptoms. You worry that you will have to start taking lots of medicines for diabetes.

You do not really know what the prostate is or does, and did not really discuss this with the last doctor. You did not discuss what the prostate test was for.

Opening statement:

'Do you have the results from the tests I had last week?'

Freely divulged in response to open questions:

Worsening LUTS for 1 year (hesitancy, weak flow, terminal dribbling).

Think symptoms due to diabetes, as your sister has been diagnosed with this and has similar symptoms.

You understand that you had tests for diabetes, your prostate and something else.

Information divulged if asked specifically:

You expect to be told that you have diabetes.

You are worried that if you have diabetes you will have to take medicines.

Last doctor mentioned that a few things could explain your symptoms including diabetes and prostate enlargement.

You did not talk much about what the prostate is, or what it does.

You did not talk much about the PSA test or interpretation of it.

You did not know that your PSA is high.

You pass urine many times during the day and night and suffer from fatigue.

You have no back pain, depression or constipation.

You want to know the implications of the PSA result; do you have cancer, are you going to die?

What happens next?

You would like an urgent referral.

NOTES

OVERALL AIM OF THE CASE

Breaking bad news and negotiating further management with the patient. The added twists here are that the patient is expecting a different bit of bad news (diabetes), and the fact that a PSA result, however high, is not a diagnostic test.

DATA GATHERING, TECHNICAL AND ASSESSMENT SKILLS

- Background to initial presentation
- Patient's understanding of what tests have been done
- Understanding of what the tests are for
- Does he know the results already?
- Clarify symptoms.

CLINICAL MANAGEMENT SKILLS

- Refer urgently to urology as a 2WW referral
- Explain that a high PSA of this order is highly suggestive of cancer but that further specialist investigations are needed to be more certain
- Outline what is likely to happen when the patient sees the urologist, ie they will offer to biopsy via the rectum and perform imaging
- Offer a follow-up appointment if any questions or concerns arise subsequently
- Suggest that he make a note of any questions that occur to him subsequently
- Offer to tell his wife with him if this is problematic for him.

INTERPERSONAL SKILLS

- Breaking bad news; have a set 'routine' that you are comfortable with
- Use a caring tone with good eye contact and open body posture
- Suggested 'stages' might include:
  - check with the patient why he thinks the tests were done
  - what has been said so far
  - give him a warning, eg 'Unfortunately I have some bad news'
  - use pauses to allow information to sink in and for the patient to ask questions
  - move at a pace dictated by the patient's responses to 'chunks' of information
  - ask the patient if he wants you to carry on
  - avoid jargon
  - empathise, eg 'I can see that you are upset by this news'
  - summarise with a clear strategy for further care
- Who can he share this information with to provide support?
- How is he getting home today and does he feel safe to make his own way home?

KEY POINTS AND FURTHER READING

NICE. *Referral guidelines for suspected cancer*, 2005. www.nice.org.uk/guidance/CG27.

NICE have produced clear guidance on 'urgent' referral under the 2-week wait rule for different suspected types of cancer. Criteria for urgent referral of urological cancer are as follows:

- Malignant-feeling prostate on digital rectal examination
- Normal feeling prostate with a high PSA for age and a life expectancy of 10+ years

CHAPTER 5

- Painless macroscopic haematuria (exclude UTI if dysuria)

- >40 years old + recurrent/persistent UTI + haematuria

- >50 years old + microscopic haematuria without proteinuria

- Masses of the renal tract identified clinically or with imaging

- Suspected penile cancer

- Swelling in the body of the testis.

NICE. *Prostate Cancer – Diagnosis and treatment*. London: NICE, 2008. www.nice.org.uk/guidance/CG58.

This guideline is primarily of interest to the urology specialist. It describes treatment algorithms for prostate cancer according to an individual's PSA level, Gleason score and staging.

NICE. *The Management of Lower Urinary Tract Symptoms in Men*. London: NICE, 2010. www.nice.org.uk/guidance/CG97.

Lower urinary tract symptoms are common complaints, especially as men get older. This guidance provides a prescriptive approach to the investigations and treatments available.

Men presenting with LUTS should be offered the following tests:

- International Prostate Symptom Score (IPSS) estimation if treatment is being considered

- Abdominal, genital and rectal examination

- Urinalysis to exclude UTI and to identify haematuria (macro-/microscopic)

- Renal function bloods and urine albumin:creatinine ratio (ACR) if renal impairment suspected

- PSA if symptoms suggest obstructive benign prostatic hypertrophy OR prostate cancer OR if the patient is concerned about prostate cancer

- Ultrasonography of renal tract if obstructive nephropathy suspected.

Men presenting with LUTS should be offered the following treatments.

- Moderate-to-severe LUTS – offer a blocker and review at 1 month, then every 6 months

- Overactive bladder – offer anticholinergic and review at 1 month, then every 6 months

- Mild LUTS and large prostate/PSA > 1.4ng/ml – offer 5a-reductase inhibitor and review at 3 months, then every 6 months

- Moderate-to-severe LUTS and large prostate/PSA > 1.4ng/ml – offer a blocker and 5a-reductase inhibitor and review at 1 month, 3 months, then every 6 months

- Storage symptoms despite a blocker – offer anticholinergic and review at 1 month then every 6 months

Consider referral to specialists in the following circumstances:

- Failed medical management for obstructive symptoms

- Urinary retention

- Suspected cancer

- Stress incontinence of urine.

Mueller PS. Breaking bad news to patients. The SPIKES approach can make this difficult task easier. *Postgrad Med* 2002;**112**(3):15–16, 18.

CHAPTER 5

This oft-cited article outlines a stepwise approach to breaking bad news using the SPIKES mnemonic:

S = setting up the interview, ie ensuring privacy. Enquire if anyone with them

P = perception, ie background to test, patient's understanding of the test

I = invitation, ie would the patient like to know the result, and how much detail?

K = knowledge, ie sharing the information, usually with a warning that it is 'bad news'

E = empathy, ie acknowledge the patient's response and emotions

S = summary, ie reiterate salient points and make a plan for follow-up.

BONUS CASE

IN THIS STATION ...

You are the duty GP at the practice.

MATERIALS AND INSTRUCTIONS TO CANDIDATE (CASE NOTES)

Name	Henry Lester
Age	68 years
Address	123a Pendred Street, Kings Cross, London
Social and family history	Tabloid photographer
	Divorced
	Lives on own
	Alcohol consumption: two bottles of wine/night
	Smoker
Past medical history	Recurrent DVT
Current medication	Warfarin 3 mg od

BRAINSTORM

EXAMINATION FINDINGS
Information offered on iPad if appropriate

Typical subconjunctival haemorrhage

BP 132/75 mmHg

INSTRUCTIONS TO THE ROLE PLAYER (PATIENT)

NOT TO BE SEEN BY THE CANDIDATE

You are Henry Lester, a 68-year-old tabloid photographer.

You're from the east end of London.

You've come to the doctor because you woke this morning with a red left eye.

You're worried about losing your eyesight and not being able to work.

Opening statement

'Hello doctor, my eye, its horrible.'

Freely divulged in response to open questions:

You woke in the morning and noticed that your eye was aching a little.

You looked in the mirror and were horrified how red it looked.

Information divulged if asked specifically:

This has never happened before.

Your vision is absolutely fine in that eye.

You don't exactly know what the INR means except that it's related to warfarin.

You haven't had your INR checked in many months; you know it's well overdue.

You haven't noticed any bleeding from elsewhere in your body.

You're not aware that alcohol can interfere with warfarin.

You know you should cut down on your drinking and shouldn't binge. You don't fully appreciate the other effects of alcohol, eg lowering of mood.

You can be lonely and feel low at times but you're not depressed. You've been banned from driving due to alcohol in the past.

You're happy to get your INR checked today and will get it done as recommended from now on.

You've been thinking of giving up smoking but haven't done anything about it.

NOTES

OVERALL AIM OF THE CASE

The aim of the case is to recognise that this patient's subconjunctival haemorrhage may be due to poorly managed warfarin. In turn, the poorly controlled warfarin could be due to alcohol abuse, as well as the patient not adhering to INR checks.

DATA GATHERING, TECHNICAL AND ASSESSMENT SKILLS

- Assessment of a red eye and establishing that it's not glaucoma, iritis, episcleritis/scleritis is a key skill.

- Questions relevant to why this patient may have had a haemorrhage are pivotal to patient safety and passing this case.

- In this case, his INR hasn't been checked for a while.

- The INR may be unstable due to his alcohol misuse; enquiring about his lifestyle will reveal the answer.

Tip

   ✓   **Asking 'why' will help you stay on track. Treating symptoms at face value without delving deeper may lead you to miss an important underlying condition.**

CLINICAL MANAGEMENT SKILLS

- His INR needs to be checked asap

- Lifestyle advice using the cycle of addiction

- Consider B vitamins and referral to local addiction service.

- Reassurance re the haemorrhage

- Appropriate safety netting.

CHAPTER 5

INTERPERSONAL SKILLS

- Understanding the patient's knowledge base is important, eg what the INR is, why monitoring INR is important, and the influence of alcohol on his mood and INR.

- Educate without being patronising.

- Don't be judgemental

KEY POINTS

- Warfarin is dangerous if the INR is not kept within range.

- Regular monitoring is essential.

- Always check that the latest INR is satisfactory before signing a script for warfarin.

- Many lifestyle factors can alter the INR including alcohol, weight change and diet.

- Check the INR after introducing or terminating a drug that may interact with warfarin.

  - Annual safety audits should be carried out in general practice (see National Patient Safety Agency for details).

REFERENCE

Thakkar R. Prescribing – Ensuring safe use of anticoagulants. *GPonline*, 2011.

CHAPTER 5

Chapter 6
Exam Circuit 3

Case Number	1	2	3	4	5	6	7	8	9	10	11	12	13
The general practice consultation	✓	✓	✓	✓	✓	✓	✓	✓	✓	✓	✓	✓	✓
Clinical governance													
Patient safety	✓	✓	✓	✓	✓	✓	✓	✓	✓	✓	✓	✓	✓
Clinical ethics and values-based practice		✓				✓					✓	✓	
Promoting equality and valuing diversity						✓					✓		
Evidence-based practice						✓							
Research and academic activity													
Teaching, mentoring and clinical supervision													
Management in primary care													
Information management and technology											✓		
Healthy people: promoting health and preventing disease	✓		✓						✓		✓		
Genetics in primary care													
Care of acutely ill people													
Care of children and young people													
Care of older adults									✓		✓		✓
Women's health			✓					✓					
Men's health								✓					
Sexual health													
Care of people with cancer and palliative care													✓
Care of people with mental health problems										✓		✓	
Care of people with learning disabilities													
Cardiovascular problems	✓				✓								
Digestive problems										✓			
Drug and alcohol problems					✓							✓	
ENT and facial problems						✓							
Eye problems													
Metabolic problems									✓				
Neurological problems										✓			
Respiratory problems	✓					✓							
Rheumatology and conditions of the musculoskeletal system (including trauma)		✓		✓							✓		
Skin problems													

Fig. 5 Circuit 3 cases plotted against RCGP curriculum

CASE 1

INSTRUCTIONS TO CANDIDATE (CASE NOTES)

You are a new GP to the practice and have never met this patient before.

Name	Richard Harris
Age	59 years
Social and family history	Married, two children
	Current smoker
Past medical history	MI and stent, 6 months ago
Current medication	Aspirin 75 mg od
	Clopidogrel 75 mg od
	Ramipril 5 mg od
	Simvastatin 40 mg nocte
	Atenolol 25 mg od

Saw the practice nurse last week for blood pressure and routine blood tests:

Recent blood pressure:	120/80 mmHg
Recent blood test:	Hb 14.9 g/dl
	Total cholesterol 4.3 mmol/l
	HDL 1.7 mmol/l

BRAINSTORM

INSTRUCTIONS TO ROLE PLAYER (PATIENT)

NOT TO BE SEEN BY THE CANDIDATE

Opening statement:

'Hello Doctor, I've been feeling breathless.'

Patient background:

You are Richard Harris, 59 years old.

You have recently gone back to work, as a foreman, after a heart attack 6 months ago. Once the doctors diagnosed your heart attack, they took you straight to a special unit where the cardiologists inserted a stent (tube-like structure) to hold open one of the arteries in your heart which was blocked.

You have been feeling breathless for about a year.

It is especially bad in the cold weather and when you exert yourself.

It is no worse at night than in the day time.

Freely divulged in response to open questions:

It is associated with a cough, productive of sputum which is sometimes green but never bloody. It tends to be productive for almost 6 months of the year.

You sometimes wheeze with it.

You continue to smoke despite your recent heart attack.

Your twin girls are at university and your wife works as the local supermarket. There is no family history of asthma.

Information divulged if asked specifically:

It is no worse laying flat in bed.

The cough is not dry or tickly.

You don't get heart burn.

There is no associated chest pain when you exert yourself. You don't experience palpitations.

You know you should give up smoking but enjoy it; you are not ready to give up at the moment.

You would rather discuss your concerns about breathlessness than smoking.

You know that smoking causes lung cancer, but you don't know about the other diseases smoking is associated with.

You take your medications as prescribed.

You did not take any medications before your heart attack. Your symptoms are no worse since starting the heart tablets.

You are concerned that you have lung cancer because you have smoked 20 a day since the age of 19. You have also been exposed to asbestos.

You are happy in yourself and enjoy life.

NOTES

OVERALL AIM OF THE CASE

Understanding what the causes of breathlessness are. Identifying a case of COPD. Respecting patient's views on their smoking habit and trying to move them along the 'cycle of change' from pre-contemplating to contemplating giving up.

DATA-GATHERING, TECHNICAL AND ASSESSMENT SKILLS

- This man is experiencing breathlessness and it is important to establish the nature of the symptoms. By reminding yourself of the possible differential diagnosis of breathlessness a focused history should be intuitive.

- Causes of breathlessness include:

  - poor conditioning

  - anaemia

  - cardiac: failure, arrhythmia, ischaemic heart disease: stent restenosis, new coronary lesions

  - respiratory: chronic obstructive pulmonary disease (COPD, this case), asthma, asbestosis, malignancy.

- Questions to consider include:

  - What does he mean by breathlessness?

  - What brings it on, moderate exertion, mild exertion, at rest, lying flat in bed? (Use the Medical Research Council [MRC] scale of breathlessness.)

  - Does he experience palpitations or exertional chest discomfort?

- Is it triggered by changes in temperature, season, stress, time of day? Does he cough or wheeze? Is the cough dry or productive?

- The patient continues to smoke which may point towards a cardiovascular or respiratory cause. Instructing him to stop smoking is counterproductive, particularly as he doesn't want to discuss smoking: respect his wishes. You may wish to ask him if he knows what the dangers of smoking are, but only if he is receptive to the discussion.

- If he did want to discuss smoking, consider the cycle of change of addiction:

The cycle of change was developed by psychologists Procheska and DiClimente. It may be applied to any patient when managing a change in behaviour, and is likely to be relevant in the mock consultation. Take smoking: a patient who already smokes may thoroughly enjoy it, may be thinking about giving up or perhaps has planned a quit programme. This being the case, if patients who are already keen to give up receive a lecture from their GP on the dangers of smoking, they may be frustrated with the care that they receive from their GP. The GP may feel that they have done their job but, in reality, they have failed. Ascertaining what the patient's views are on smoking is a good way of gauging where they are in the cycle of change. That way, the patient can be helped and will feel listened to.

CHAPTER 6

1. Precontemplation – patient enjoying behaviour, little motivation to change – eating too much, smoking etc. The doctor's role is to get the patient thinking that changing their behaviour would be in their health interests to do so. This may move the patient on to the contemplation stage.

2. Contemplation – patient thinking they should give up the behaviour but haven't planned how to go about it.

3. Planning – active management plan to give up the behaviour, eg smoking counselling, commence nicotine replacement, phased reduction in number of cigarettes smoked.

4. Action – quit date.

5. Maintenance – period of time patient abstains from behaviour.

6. Relapse – patient resumes behaviour, may enter cycle at stage 1, 2 or 3.

Reprinted from *GP ST: Stage 3 Assessment Handbook* Raj Thakkar (2008).

- He has smoked 20 cigarettes a day for 40 years = 40 pack-years.

- The history points toward a diagnosis of COPD: he has a productive cough and wheeze without cardiac symptoms. If he had a dry cough, ramipril may be implicated. If he had wheeze without sputum production and his symptoms had started after he was commenced on cardiac drugs, atenolol may have been implicated in causing bronchospasm.

- Examination of both the cardiovascular and respiratory systems is appropriate. Consider re-checking his blood pressure; 120/80 seems a bit too good to be true! The examiners will not be expecting an MRCGP-perfect systems-based examination; they will be more impressed if you perform a focused examination relevant to the patient. It would be appropriate to examine him on the couch, top exposed if he is agreeable. Check his pulse, blood pressure, feel his cardiac apex, percuss for effusions, and listen to his heart and breath sounds. Checking for conjunctival pallor is reasonable given that he is breathless. Examination should be slick and shouldn't take long.

Tip

   ✓   **Practise your examination skills before the CSA until you are slick and efficient.**

- If you have time, consider whether he has depression after his myocardial infarction and be sensitive when discussing the possibility of another chronic disease, eg COPD. Some data suggest that 90% of patients with COPD have depression.

CLINICAL MANAGEMENT SKILLS

- Smoking cessation: most practices offer or have access to smoking cession clinics. He isn't keen to discuss smoking today but he may change his mind.

- His diagnosis is likely to be COPD, but you need to confirm the diagnosis. It is important to refer him to the practice nurse for spirometry. Most practices will have a spirometer; given that the Quality and Outcomes Framework (QOF) rewards its use. Reversibility testing is included in the QOF to help exclude asthma.

- Given his exposure to cigarette smoke as well as asbestos, it would be reasonable to organise a chest radiograph.

- Organising a full blood count may be appropriate as he is breathless, to ensure that he is not anaemic, particularly as he is on aspirin and clopidogrel.

- You may consider starting him on a short-acting β agonist (SABA) in the first instance and advise him to see the practice nurse to teach him how to use it.

INTERPERSONAL SKILLS

- Breathlessness is a frightening experience. It is important to make him feel at ease and free to express his fears.

CHAPTER 6

- Remember, until he has had formal spirometry, it wouldn't be wise to give him a formal diagnosis of COPD. You may however, introduce the idea of him having a smoking-related disease. How would you do this? You may ask if knows anyone else with smoking-related lung problems.

- Offer to discuss smoking if he so wishes; be explicit. Discuss it without being patronising, but only if he wishes to do so. By explaining the risks of smoking, you may encourage him to give up. He may want to attend a smoking cessation clinic. Would he prefer nicotine replacement therapy or alternative treatments rather than attend a dedicated clinic? If he doesn't want to use the clinic, why not, what are his fears?

- How will you explain what COPD is? Perhaps use visual aids or suggest that he looks at a website such as www.patient.co.uk

- What are his concerns? This patient is concerned about lung cancer and has little idea about COPD. How can you reassure him; how would he like to be reassured: a chest radiograph, for example?

- Once a discussion has taken place about the possibility of COPD, negotiate whether he is happy to have appropriate investigations. He may not want to; perhaps he would rather have a chest radiograph, perhaps give up smoking and then see if his symptoms improve.

- Does he know what spirometry is?

- He may ask about treatment of COPD, despite not having confirmatory tests as yet. If you are running out of time it is appropriate to apologise and suggest, if he wouldn't mind, talking through the treatment if the diagnosis is confirmed.

- Appropriate follow-up is required to provide further encouragement in smoking cessation and to follow up results of investigations and to formulate any treatment strategies.

- Safety-netting is required to seek advice if he becomes acutely breathless.

CHAPTER 6

SMOKING CESSATION TREATMENT OPTIONS

	BUPROPION	NICOTINE	VARENICLINE
BRAND	Zyban	Nicorette Nicotinell NiquItin Niquitin CQ	Champix
PRESENTATION	Prolonged release, film-coated tablets	Gum Inhalator (Nicorette only) Lozenges Microtabs (Nicorette only) Nasal spray (Nicorette only) Transdermal patches	Film-coated tablets
TREATMENT DURATION	7–9 weeks	10–12 weeks	12 weeks
CONTRAINDICATIONS	• History of seizures • CNS tumour • Bulimia, anorexia nervosa • Bipolar disorder • Severe hepatic cirrhosis • Patients experiencing abrupt withdrawal of alcohol or benzodiazepines	None	None
USE IN PREGNANCY	No	Yes • Intermittent dosing products are preferable as they provide lower daily dose of nicotine • Patches may be preferred if woman suffering from nausea • Patches should be removed before going to bed • Aim to discontinue after 2–3 months	No
USE IN LACTATION	No	Yes • Intermittent dosing products are preferable	No
RECOMMENDED BY NICE	Yes	Yes	Yes
MODE OF ACTION	Inhibits the reuptake of noradrenaline and dopamine resulting in a reduction in craving and withdrawal symptoms.	Nicotine replacement therapy allows the psychological addition of the smoking habit to be dealt with separately from the physical addiction to nicotine.	Binds nicotine acetylcholine receptors to alleviate symptoms of craving and withdrawal. Also competes with nicotine at the receptor binding sites, resulting in a reduction of the rewarding and reinforcing effects of smoking.

• All smokers should be advised to stop and offered help if interested in doing so.

• Smoking cessation therapies should be offered when appropriate, and where possible, smokers should have access to a smoking cessation clinic or programme for behavioural support.

CHAPTER 6

Fig. 6 Smoking cessation treatment options

Reproduced with the kind permission of MIMS

KEY POINTS AND FURTHER READING

NOTES ON COPD

NICE. *Management of COPD in adults in primary and secondary care*. London: NICE, 2010. www.nice.org.uk/guidance/CG101

- Consider diagnosis in:
  - those over 35 years old who are current smokers, ex-smokers or have other risk factors
  - those with a history of chronic cough, wheeze, regular sputum production and exertional breathlessness
  - those who have bronchitis occurring frequently in winter.
- Spirometry with reversibility testing should be offered
- $FEV_1/FVC < 0.7$
- Mild COPD: FEV_1 >80% of predicted
- Moderate COPD: FEV_1 50–79% of predicted
- Severe COPD: FEV_1 30–49% of predicted
- Very severe COPD: FEV_1 <30%
- Consider asthma if > 400 ml (FEV_1) response to bronchodilators/ prednisolone trial
- All patients should be educated: smoking cessation advice; influenza vaccination
- Patients should be offered maintenance treatment if they are breathless or have exacerbations despite treatment with short-acting inhaled drugs:
  - If FEV_1 > 50% predicted, offer long-acting β agonists (LABAs) or long-acting anticholinergics (LAMAs)
  - If FEV_1 < 50% predicted, offer either combination LABA and ICS inhaler, or LAMA
  - If breathlessness or patient continues to have exacerbations despite LABA and ICS, add in LAMA irrespective of FEV_1.
- Consider pulmonary rehabilitation including for those who have had a recent hospitalisation.

CHAPTER 6

CASE 2

INSTRUCTIONS TO CANDIDATES (CASE NOTES)

You are a locum GP and have never worked in the practice before.

Name	Rose Shanahan
Age	62 years
Social and family history	Lives with husband
Past medical history	Osteoarthritis
	Total knee replacement: 3 weeks ago
	Hypertension
Current medication	Cocodamol 30/500 max 2 qds
	Amlodipine 5mg od

Saw the practice nurse this morning for blood pressure and routine blood tests:

Blood pressure this am	136/78 mmHg

BRAINSTORM

INSTRUCTIONS TO ROLE PLAYER (PATIENT)

NOT TO BE SEEN BY THE CANDIDATE

Patient background:

You are 62-year-old Rose Shanahan.

You had a total knee replacement of your right knee 3 weeks ago.

You are not happy with it and would like a second opinion to see if it was done properly.

It is still painful.

Opening statement:

'Hi Doctor, I want a second opinion.'

Freely divulged in response to open questions:

You're sorry to make a fuss.

Your knee continues to be in pain, the pain is throbbing in nature.

You had a recent knee replacement.

Information divulged if asked specifically:

You were expecting it to be pain free by now.

You can't remember exactly what the surgeon and physiotherapist told you about recovery and you lost the post-surgery information sheet.

You are keen to get back to dancing.

It has been warm and swollen since the operation. The swelling is less than it was last week.

You have not felt feverish.

The wound is looking clean and it hasn't oozed any pus.

Admittedly it has been getting less painful as time goes by.

You want to drive; it is important as you have a disabled grandchild who needs to be taken to his therapy group while your daughter is at work.

CHAPTER 6

You don't like pills and only take 1 co-codamol (30/500) tablet at night.

You're embarrassed to say that the co-codamol made you constipated, you have not suffered any weight loss or gain, and you have never seen any blood in the stool.

You have never had a stomach ulcer and have never had problems with ibuprofen. You are not asthmatic.

NOTES

OVERALL AIM OF THE CASE

To identify the patient's expectations, which were unrealistic in terms of healing, and to avoid the need for an unnecessary referral.

DATA-GATHERING, TECHNICAL AND ASSESSMENT SKILLS

- Establishing what the patient was told by the hospital is important.
- Was she given any leaflets by the hospital and has she read them?
- You should ask about and examine, unless the patient declines, to exclude complications of knee replacement, eg DVT, infection, peroneal nerve palsy, vascular complications.
- Has she tried to drive so far?
- What analgesia is she taking?
- Does she have any side effects from her medication; does she know what side effects she may expect?
- Perhaps consider other causes of constipation; does she have any features of hypothyroidism, has she noticed any red flag symptoms suggestive of bowel cancer?

CHAPTER 6

CLINICAL MANAGEMENT SKILLS

- Offer alternative analgesia.

- Offer laxatives.

- If you have a high index of suspicion for infection or DVT, she should be referred to secondary care for assessment.

INTERPERSONAL SKILLS

- This consultation is partly about managing the patient's expectations.

- Does she know how long it takes most people to recover? Swimming can commence once the wound has healed. Non-stressful activities, including dancing, can commence around 6 weeks whereas activities that stress the joint should be avoided, eg squash.

- Does she know anyone else who may have had a knee replacement? How long did they take to fully recover? In general, patients may take 2 months before they return to work.

- What does she hope another surgeon would do at this early stage?

- Does she have any particular concerns that you may be able to address?

- Try to get her to realise why driving may be dangerous, perhaps by asking her if she knows what the risks are. If she can't see why driving may be dangerous, perhaps offer an example, eg inability to perform an emergency stop. Driving may commence as soon as 1 week after left knee replacement but may be 4–6 weeks after right knee replacement.

- Explore why she is not keen to take her analgesia. Can you offer her options (eg paracetamol, non-steroidal anti-inflammatory drugs [NSAIDS]) and agree a plan that suits her. You will need to discuss the pros and cons of each option so that she can make an informed choice.

CHAPTER 6

- Reiterate the complications of having knee replacement, and check you understand her and she understands you.

- Share a management plan together and agree a reasonable follow-up appointment.

FURTHER READING

Detailed notes on 'Knee Joint Replacements – What a GP Needs to Know' are produced by www.patient.co.uk.

Also knee replacement surgery: www.arthritisresearchuk.org/arthritis-information/surgery/knee-replacement.aspx

CASE 3

INSTRUCTIONS TO CANDIDATES (CASE NOTES)

You are a locum GP and have never worked in the practice before.

Name   Sarah Jones

Age   59 years

The patient is new to the surgery and her notes have not been summarised on to the computer records.

BRAINSTORM

Tip

✓ In the examination, there may be cases where you have little information to brainstorm points that you would like to bring up. If so, take a breather and compose yourself or remind yourself of consultation styles and techniques.

INSTRUCTIONS TO ROLE PLAYER (PATIENT)

NOT TO BE SEEN BY THE CANDIDATE

Patient background:

Your name is Sarah Jones, you are 59 years old.

You are a headmistress and have recently moved to the local area.

You first ask for a repeat prescription of your blood pressure tablets (amlodipine 5 mg) which you've been on for 2 years. Your blood pressure has always been well controlled on this drug and you only had it checked last week by your old GP who said it was 135/70. You appear distracted and, if the doctor doesn't ask if there is something worrying you, you allude (through non-verbal cues) to there being something else that you would like to discuss – something 'embarrassing'. You do admit that there is something embarrassing that you'd like to discuss; you do this early in the consultation.

You live with your husband and don't have children (through choice).

Your hidden agenda is to discuss vaginal bleeding. YOU DECLINE AN EXAMINATION IF OFFERED but accept a referral to a gynaecologist.

Opening statement:

'Hello, I was wondering if I could have some more of my tablets' (you have an empty box of your old tablets).

CHAPTER 6

Freely divulged in response to open questions:

You have never smoked and have a very healthy diet.

You exercise regularly.

Your GP recently checked your cholesterol which was excellent but you can't remember the number.

He also checked to see if you were diabetic, which you're not.

Both your parents had strokes in their 80s.

Your mother had endometrial (womb) cancer.

You have experienced vaginal spotting (fresh blood) for 4 months.

It has been getting heavier lately and you are now bleeding on a daily basis.

You do not want an intimate examination today.

You would like to be referred to a female gynaecologist for further investigation.

Information divulged if asked specifically:

Your best friend urged you to see the doctor.

You sometimes pass blood clots.

You're sexually active and faithful to your partner.

Bleeding isn't provoked by intercourse.

You don't have any pelvic pain.

Your last smear, 2 years ago, was normal.

You had the menopause at age 53.

You have felt more tired lately.

You have been frightened in case you have womb cancer, as your mother had.

You have not been experiencing bloating or breathlessness.

NOTES

OVERALL AIM OF THE CASE

This case aims to establish the patient's hidden agenda, which is to discuss vaginal bleeding. It then tests the candidate's ability to manage a potentially serious clinical condition while addressing the patient's concerns.

DATA-GATHERING, TECHNICAL AND ASSESSMENT SKILLS

• It is important to take a brief history regarding high blood pressure. How long has she had it for? Does she have any other cardiovascular risk factors? It is sometimes difficult to take over the care of a chronic disease in a new patient. In some situations, there may be good reason to double-check the patient's blood pressure again. In this case it is useful to have her blood pressure on your record, especially as you are responsible for the drug that you are going to prescribe. In addition, this will satisfy the QOF requirement.

• Postmenopausal bleeding (PMB) should be taken seriously as it may be a sign of malignancy.

• It is generally accepted that bleeding 12 months after the last menstrual period is considered postmenopausal.

• Ten per cent of women with PMB will have endometrial carcinoma. It is important to consider when the bleeding started, the approximate volume of blood loss and when it happens. Smear history is relevant in case the bleeding is cervical in origin.

• Risk factors for endometrial carcinoma should be part of the history and includes; age (peak age approx 60), obesity, parity (higher incidence in nulliparous women), late menopause, diabetes, unopposed oestrogen (which is why hormone replacement therapy [HRT] should include cyclical progestogen in women who have not

CHAPTER 6

263

had a hysterectomy), and family history (including a family history of hereditary non-polyposis colorectal cancer). In premenopausal women, irregular or heavy periods may be the presenting feature.

- Tamoxifen increases the risk of endometrial carcinoma.

- HRT complicates the clinical picture. If patients are on HRT, bleeding may also be caused by poor compliance or poor absorption. One should enquire if the bleeding is cyclical and if she is taking other medications (which can interact).

- Examination of the abdomen wouldn't be unreasonable to check for a bulky uterus and evidence of metastatic disease.

Tip

   ✓   **For the purposes of this examination, intimate examinations are not permitted. However, you should express to the examiner that you would consider performing such an examination and why.**

- Her tiredness is likely to be secondary to anaemia. It would be reasonable to consider whether anaemia has caused cardio-respiratory compromise.

CLINICAL MANAGEMENT SKILLS

- She should be given a repeat prescription for amlodipine and arrange follow-up.

- This patient may have a gynaecological malignancy. She has a number of risk factors for endometrial cancer and she should be referred to the gynaecology team on a 2-week-wait (2WW) basis.

- She is feeling tired and it is likely that the bleeding has led to anaemia. Organising an FBC is entirely appropriate.

CHAPTER 6

INTERPERSONAL SKILLS

- PMB is a clearly a sensitive issue for her and one should be aware of this.

- She is obviously embarrassed and very worried; make her feel at ease. Non-verbal cues may be used, for example: 'You look very worried … you seem to have something on your mind … are you ok? You seem troubled …'

- Check that you understand exactly what the history is, perhaps by summarising the history back to her.

- Consider what her fears are: cancer (given her mother had endometrial cancer too). If you are aware what her fears are, she will be satisfied you are taking them into account in your management. What was her experience with her mother?

- Introducing the idea that PMB may have a sinister aetiology is required to agree a management plan. This must be done in a sensitive manner, perhaps by asking her what she thinks may be the cause of the bleeding, how her mum presented or what her concerns are. In this way, the discussion can be based around her own health beliefs.

- A management plan should be agreed by you both (shared management).

- She should be appropriately followed up: to ensure that she has had her blood tests and to discuss the results with her, to ensure that she has received an appointment from the gynaecologist, and that she has indeed attended. She may also want to come back in case she has more questions; she should know this opportunity is available.

CHAPTER 6

CASE 4

INSTRUCTIONS TO CANDIDATES (CASE NOTES)

You are a locum GP and have never worked in the practice before.

Name	Petra Lipinski
Age	62 years
Social and family history	Lives with partner
	Language teacher
Past medical history	Appendicectomy, 2001
	Hypertension
	Osteoarthritis, knees
Current medication	Ramipril 5 mg od
	Co-codamol, 30/500 max 2 qds
Allergies	NSAIDs
	Amlodipine
Last consultation (2 months ago):	
	BP 123/80
	BMI 22

Left knee pain continues – not locking; injected with 80 mg methylprednisolone, aseptic technique. Medial approach. Warned re infections. Review if concerned; otherwise repeat injection in 6 months.

BRAINSTORM

INSTRUCTIONS TO ROLE PLAYER (PATIENT)

NOT TO BE SEEN BY THE CANDIDATE

Patient background:

You are Petra Lipinski, a 62-year-old teacher.

You have been in the UK for 30 years.

You have had high blood pressure for 10 years which has always been well controlled on ramipril.

You have osteoarthritis in both knees from your days as a runner.

Your arthritis was formally diagnosed 15 years ago by X-ray.

You're not keen on a clinical examination today.

Opening statement:

'My knee is playing up again doctor'

Freely divulged in response to open questions:

Your left knee has always been the one that has caused you the most pain.

You're aware the X-ray of the left knee revealed more advanced arthritis than the right.

Your right knee has never caused you any problems.

You take co-codamol 30/500, two tablets, four times a day to help with pain in your left knee.

You have steroid injections twice a year to help with the pain.

Information divulged if asked specifically:

You can't quite remember exactly what osteoarthritis is. You think it is when the joints get damaged.

You buy lactulose syrup to help with constipation, which you always get with codeine.

You can't take any drugs like ibuprofen; they all cause a rash.

The injections normally help but your knee has become painful only 2 months after your previous injection.

You don't exercise and have never tried physiotherapy or acupuncture.

You have never tried glucosamine, although you have heard of it.

The knee doesn't give way or lock.

It is impacting on your quality of life and causes you pain on a daily basis, especially whenever you are on your feet.

You are often in pain at work and sometimes have to teach sitting down. Your headmaster doesn't mind and he is very supportive.

You find the pain distracting during lesson times.

You are able to wash and dress yourself.

Stairs can be painful and you sometimes have to take short steps to reduce the pain.

All of your other joints are fine.

You are not unhappy in yourself.

You are happy to try physiotherapy and swimming.

You would rather not have stronger pain-killers at this stage.

You would consider taking glucosamine, but you're not sure where to get it from.

You may consider acupuncture.

You don't want to be referred to an orthopaedic surgeon; you are fearful of having a knee replacement. You know someone who recently had a replacement and they are in constant pain.

You're happy to try out some of the therapies discussed and review the situation in a few months.

CHAPTER 6

NOTES

OVERALL AIM OF THE CASE

This case discusses the patient with advanced knee arthritis who does not want a knee replacement but is willing to try alternative therapies.

NICE published guidelines on osteoarthritis in February 2008. The important points have been incorporated into these notes.

DATA-GATHERING, TECHNICAL AND ASSESSMENT SKILLS

- Important features to consider with knee pain include:
  - the background to the condition – when was it diagnosed, how did she get it (eg running – as in this case, sport, accident, septic joint)
  - are other joints are affected?
  - treatment so far? – drugs (over the counter and prescribed), physiotherapy, acupuncture, joint injection with steroid
  - treatments that have worked
  - impact on her quality of life – home and work
  - is it making her unhappy?
  - does the knee give way or lock? If so, under what circumstances?
- Examination of the knee should ideally be done on the couch. Remember – look, feel, move, function. You should look for deformity and scars, palpate for joint-line tenderness and crepitus, assess range of movement, and check for laxity of the collateral and cruciate ligaments. Asking her to walk may reveal an antalgic gait.

CLINICAL MANAGEMENT SKILLS

- Consider:
  - holistic approach
  - educate patient on osteoarthritis (OA)

CHAPTER 6

- encourage exercise
- sensible footwear
- heat/cold packs
- transcutaneous electrical nerve stimulation (TENS) machine
- analgesia
- topical capsaicin
- intra-articular steroid injections
- physiotherapy/occupational therapy
- glucosamine not advised by NICE – however, Gait trial, 2006, showed statistically significant benefit
- referral for arthroscopic lavage/debridement shouldn't be offered unless knee locking
- referral for surgery if symptoms have substantial impact on quality of life and if non-surgical treatments have failed.

INTERPERSONAL SKILLS

- Consider what the patient's thoughts are; does she know what osteoarthritis actually is?
- Is she aware how she may have developed it?
- What are her concerns? eg knee replacement, disability.
- What are her expectations? What does she hope to achieve from treatments? Does she know what the side effects may be?
- Share management options, let her know what options are available to her, giving pros and cons and help her choose a strategy that is acceptable to her.
- Agree suitable follow-up.

FURTHER READING

www.nice.org.uk (see document CG59)

www.arthritisresearchuk.org

CASE 5

INSTRUCTIONS TO CANDIDATES (CASE NOTES)

You are a locum GP and have never worked in the practice before.

Name	Mr Rizwan Patel
Occupation	Economics teacher
Age	51 years
Family history	Father MI
	Mother CVA
Social history	Originally from south Asia
	Married, three children
Past medical history	Obesity
	Hypercholesterolaemia
Current medication	Atorvastatin 40 mg nocte

Saw the practice nurse last week for blood pressure and routine blood tests:

Recent blood pressures
(taken on three separate occasions by the nurse)

175/93, 172/97, 165/96 mmHg

Recent blood tests   Total cholesterol 4.8 mmol/l

HDL 0.9 mmol/l

eGFR > 90 ml/min

BRAINSTORM

INSTRUCTIONS TO ROLE PLAYER (PATIENT)

NOT TO BE SEEN BY THE CANDIDATE

Patient background:

Your name is Rizwan Patel, you are 51 years old.

You have been seeing the practice nurse over the past month for blood pressure (BP) checks. It has been consistently high and she has asked you to see the doctor.

You have a history of high cholesterol which runs in your family. You take a cholesterol tablet for this (atorvastatin 40 mg).

You take your medication every day without fail.

Opening statement:

'Hello Doctor! I've been told to see you by the nurse. My blood pressure is too high!'

Freely divulged in response to open questions:

You are unsure why treating blood pressure is important, although you are willing to take any medication that the doctor suggests.

You wonder what you can do to reduce your blood pressure yourself. You don't mind taking tablets in the meantime until you can alter your lifestyle.

You know you are overweight and don't look after your diet.

Information divulged if asked specifically:

You are not quite sure what blood pressure means, in particular you would like to know what the ideal BP is and what the significance of each number is.

You drink 2 × 250 ml glasses of (12%) wine per night. You sometimes don't drink any alcohol at all, but two glasses is the norm. You never drink in the mornings. Last week, you went away for a city break and didn't drink at all.

You don't exercise although you know that you should.

When you do exert yourself you do not experience any chest discomfort.

You have never smoked.

You don't have to get up in the night to pass urine and don't complain of excessive thirst or tiredness.

NOTES

OVERALL AIM OF THE CASE

The aim of this case is to demonstrate proficient management of high blood pressure, a common case in general practice.

DATA-GATHERING, TECHNICAL AND ASSESSMENT SKILLS

- This patient is at risk of cardiovascular disease because of his ethnicity, hypertension, requirement to take statins and obesity.

- His blood pressure should be re-checked in order to confirm that it is high. (The examiner may tell you what today's reading is.)

- It is important to consider risk factors for hypertension; these include obesity and alcohol. His weight should be measured.

- For the examination, weighing him without shoes and debris in his pockets is sufficient. You may say to him that you will document that he was weighed with his clothes on but without shoes.

- His weekly alcohol consumption should be calculated using his daily consumption:

  - (ml)/1000 × % alcohol = 500/1000 × 12 = 6 units.

  - Therefore his weekly consumption is: 6 × 7 = 42 units.

- One should sensitively establish whether he is dependent on alcohol.

- Other cardiovascular risk factors should be discussed and checked, including smoking status and family history.

- It would be prudent to establish whether he has symptoms suggestive of coronary artery disease: exertional chest pain and breathlessness.

- A cardiovascular examination is important, in part, to establish whether there are any signs of aortic stenosis if you are considering prescribing ACE-inhibitors (ACEIs).

Tip

    ✓   **You should not expect to find any abnormal signs during the CSA. If you do, it is likely to be by chance.**

- This patient may be diabetic and you should ask about symptoms suggestive of hyperglycaemia.

CLINICAL MANAGEMENT SKILLS

- A discussion about lifestyle should take place.

- Advise that addressing his lifestyle issues may eliminate the need for blood pressure medication which may provide an added incentive to lose weight and reduce his alcohol intake.

- According to the cycle of change of addiction, if he already realises that he wants to address lifestyle issues, your time is better spent discussing how he can reduce his weight and alcohol consumption. Of course, if he is resistant to this perhaps discussing the risks of not addressing lifestyle and the benefits of doing so would be appropriate.

- Ideally he should cut down on alcohol, improve his diet and exercise more.

- He should be encouraged to lose around 1–2 pounds (approx. 0.5–1 kg)/week of weight by diet and exercise. This could be monitored by the practice health care assistant (HCA).

- You should offer ambulatory blood pressure monitoring (ABPM) to confirm the diagnosis of hypertension as per NICE guidelines. If there is severe hypertension consider starting treatment immediately without waiting for results of ABPM.

- As he is aged <55 he should be commenced on an ACE inhibitor. He should be warned about the side effects as detailed in the *British National Formulary* (BNF) – including first-dose hypotension, cough and angio-oedema.

- His eGFR creatinine should be monitored around 10 days after commencement of an ACEI (explain why). After his blood test, you should review him to discuss the result and re-check his blood

CHAPTER 6

pressure. If his blood pressure is not controlled the dose could be increased and his eGFR creatinine re-checked accordingly.

- He should be warned that he may need higher doses of the drug and more than one drug may be required (he will therefore know what to expect).

Tip

> ✓ **Don't be reluctant to use your BNF in the CSA.**

- His blood glucose should be checked.

INTERPERSONAL SKILLS

- Discussing a patient's lifestyle, including weight and alcohol consumption, is not always easy and it should be done sensitively. One way around this would be to ask him about what he thinks about his own lifestyle and the effects that it may have on his health (his ideas). If prompting is required, you could give some of the factors that contribute to high blood pressure; include alcohol and being overweight. He may then offer his sentiments regarding both of these.

- What are his ideas on the causes of cardiovascular disease?

- It is important to get him on board with lifestyle changes.

- Education and regular follow-up are both important in this case. He has a number of questions and he should be given the opportunity to ask these and any concerns that he has.

- Managing his expectations may improve his adherence to medication and maintain his satisfaction. Many patients don't realise that they may have to stay on blood pressure medication permanently (around 70% of patients will remain on antihypertensive drugs), and few realise that the initial dose may not be sufficient to control it. Explain that he may need to go on higher-dose medication and more than one drug if the initial dose that you prescribed doesn't control his blood pressure.

- Without explanation, patients may think that they need to take only a one-month course as prescribed.

CHAPTER 6

Clinical Management of Primary Hypertension in Adults NICE Guideline

Measurement
- If BP ≥140/90mmHg, take a second reading; if considerably different, take a third. Record the lower of the last two measurements as clinic BP.
- Take a supine or seated reading in patients with symptoms of postural hypotension, followed by a reading after ≥1 min standing.
- If clinic BP is ≥140/90mmHg, offer ambulatory blood pressure monitoring (ABPM) to confirm diagnosis.
- If patient is unable to tolerate ABPM, offer home blood pressure monitoring (HBPM).
- If severe hypertension, consider starting treatment immediately without waiting for results of ABPM or HBPM.
- Measure BP on both of patient's arms, if difference is >20mmHg repeat the measurement and if it remains >20mmHg use the arm with the higher reading for future measurements.
- While waiting for ABPM or HBPM results, test for proteinuria. Measure plasma glucose, electrolytes, creatinine, eGFR, serum total cholesterol and HDL-cholesterol. Arrange a 12-lead ECG. Assess for hypertensive retinopathy.
- Estimate 10-year cardiovascular disease (CVD) risk in accordance with the Joint British Societies assessment scheme www.bhsoc.org.
- If hypertension is not diagnosed, assess in 5 years or consider more frequently if clinic BP is close to 140/90mmHg.

ABPM
- Take ≥2 measurements per hour during patient's usual waking hours.
- Use average value of ≥14 measurements to confirm diagnosis.

HBPM
- For each BP recording, take two measurements ≥1 min apart whilst patient is seated.
- Record BP twice daily, ideally in the morning and evening.
- Record BP for ≥4 days, ideally 7 days.
- Discard measurements on day 1 and use the average value of remaining measurements to confirm diagnosis.

Aims
- To reduce clinic BP to <140/90mmHg or average ABPM/HBPM to <135/85mmHg in patients <80 years.
- To reduce clinic BP to <150/90mmHg or average ABPM/HBPM to <145/85mmHg in patients ≥80 years.

Note: See Hypertension in Pregnancy (NICE CG 107) for advice on the management of hypertension in women of childbearing potential.

	Clinic BP (mmHg)		Average ABPM or HBPM (mmHg)	Recommended Action
Stage 1 hypertension	≥140/90	and	≥135/85	Offer treatment to patients <80 years with ≥1 of the following: target organ damage, established CVD, renal disease, diabetes or a 10 year CVD risk ≥20%.
Stage 2 hypertension	≥160/100	and	≥150/95	Offer treatment to patients of any age.
Severe hypertension	systolic ≥180 or diastolic ≥110		-	Consider immediate treatment.

Lifestyle measures
- Offer lifestyle advice to all patients undergoing assessment or treatment for hypertension.
- Assess patients' diet and exercise patterns and encourage appropriate lifestyle changes.
- Advise patients to:
- – Limit weekly alcohol intake.
- – Avoid excessive consumption of coffee and other caffeine-rich products.
- – Limit dietary sodium intake by reducing intake or substituting sodium salt.
- Offer smoking cessation help and advice.
- Encourage stress reduction.

Note: Calcium, magnesium or potassium supplements should not be offered as a method for reducing BP.

Treatment
- Offer patients ≥80 years the same treatment as younger patients taking account of any co-morbidity and patient's existing burden of drug use.
- Offer patients with isolated systolic hypertension (systolic BP ≥160mmHg) the same treatment as patients with both raised systolic and diastolic BP.
- Provide patients with appropriate guidance and material about the benefits of drugs and the unwanted side effects that may occur in order to help patients make informed choices.
- Where possible, recommend treatment with drugs that can be taken once daily.
- Prescribe generic preparations where these are appropriate and minimise cost.
- Use clinic BP measurements to monitor response to treatment. Consider ABPM or HBPM as an adjunct in patients identified as having 'white-coat effect'.

Continued on the following page

CHAPTER 6

Management of Hypertension *continued*

TREATMENT ALGORITHM

A = ACE inhibitor (or angiotensin II receptor antagonist if ACE inhibitor not tolerated)
C = Calcium-channel blocker
D = Thiazide-like diuretic eg, chlortalidone or indapamide

Note
– β-blockers are not a preferred initial therapy but are an alternative in patients <55 years with an intolerance or contraindication to ACE inhibitors (or angiotensin II receptor antagonists), women of childbearing potential, or if evidence of increased sympathetic drive.
– If therapy initiated with a β-blocker, add a calcium-channel blocker rather than a thiazide-like diuretic to reduce risk of diabetes.
– In patients well controlled with a regimen that includes a conventional thiazide diuretic, there is no absolute need to replace the conventional thiazide diuretic with an alternative agent.
– If calcium-channel blocker not suitable or not tolerated, offer thiazide-like diuretic.
– Angiotensin II receptor antagonist preferred to ACE inhibitor in black patients of African/Caribbean descent.

Follow-up
● Annual review – monitor BP, provide patients with support and discuss lifestyle, symptoms and medication.

Specialist referral
● Consider in patients with signs and symptoms suggesting secondary cause of hypertension. Accelerated (malignant) hypertension or suspected phaeochromocytoma require immediate referral.
● Consider in patients with symptoms of, or documented, postural hypotension (fall in systolic BP when standing of 20mmHg or more).
● Consider in patients with unusual signs or symptoms or in those whose management depends critically on the accurate measurement of their BP.
● Consider if <40 years and no evidence of target organ damage, CVD, renal disease or diabetes.

Adapted from: NICE Clinical Guideline 127 (August 2011) · Hypertension: clinical management of primary hypertension in adults (partially updates and replaces NICE Clinical Guideline 34). The full NICE guideline is available at www.nice.org.uk. A quick reference guide is also available.

CHAPTER 6

Fig. 7 Clinical management of primary hypertension in adults, NICE guidelines

Reproduced with the kind permission of MIMS

CASE 6

INSTRUCTIONS TO CANDIDATES (CASE NOTES)

You are a locum GP and have never worked in the practice before.

Name	Peter Hendry
Age	52 years
Social and family history	Married, four children
Past medical history	Osteoarthritis
	Hypercholesterolaemia
Current medication	Paracetamol 500 mg prn
	Simvastatin 40 mg nocte

Saw the practice nurse 2 weeks ago for blood pressure and routine blood tests:

Recent blood pressure	137/82 mmHg
Recent blood tests	Hb 14.9 g/dl
	Total cholesterol 3.9 mmol/l
	HDL 1.9 mmol/l
	BMI 30

BRAINSTORM

INSTRUCTIONS TO ROLE PLAYER (PATIENT)

NOT TO BE SEEN BY THE CANDIDATE

Patient background:

You are Peter Hendry, a 52-year-old director of a plumbing firm.

You are waving a newspaper article.

You have a copy of today's tabloid newspaper.

You highlight an article on statins. The article deems simvastatin an old drug with many side effects.

A new statin, Gold XR, was reviewed in the article. It has been on the market for a week now. A major medical trial, run by the drug company that manufacture Gold XR, concluded that all patients should be switched to the new wonder drug. They claim that the drug can reduce deaths from heart disease, stroke, and Alzheimer's disease by 50%.

You are surprised that the doctor hasn't heard of the drug.

You would like to have the new statin rather than simvastatin.

Opening statement:

'Hi Doctor, I'd like to change my cholesterol tablets!'

Freely divulged in response to open questions:

You think that if the government can pay for polyclinics, there must be millions of pounds in the pot.

You feel that you are entitled to the best possible treatment on the NHS as you have paid your taxes.

You don't particularly look after your diet and you don't exercise.

You say you smoke a little.

Information divulged if asked specifically:

You admit to smoking 25 cigarettes a day; you enjoy smoking.

You don't realise that some patients have had to pay for their own chemotherapy – such is the state of the NHS.

CHAPTER 6

You have no idea that the government is squeezing the NHS so much that patients are being refused surgery, eg for varicose veins and hernias.

You hadn't considered that, if the study is sponsored by the drug company, there may be a biased slant to the story.

You are embarrassed as you didn't even think that the newspaper would sensationalise a major health topic.

You think 50% improvement is a massive improvement.

You take statins so you don't have to exercise so much and can continue your current unhealthy lifestyle.

NOTES

OVERALL AIM OF THE CASE

This case is challenging, requiring the candidate to establish the patient's understanding and thought process, and educate him with a view to changing his agenda.

DATA-GATHERING, TECHNICAL AND ASSESSMENT SKILLS

- Consider why he requires statins in the first place; in this case it is likely to be a substitute for not exercising and having a poor diet.

- Why does he want to have Gold XL in particular?

- What are his views on his recent cholesterol results? Does he know what they mean?

- What are his views on his lifestyle? Does he think that he should change?

- How does he feel about smoking?

CHAPTER 6

- Find out if he knows the about the dangers of smoking (to try to change his view from pre-contemplation to contemplation).

- What are his views on the press and how and why it delivers stories?

- A discussion about what 50% reduction in heart disease, stroke and Alzheimer's disease actually means should take place, first by asking him what he thinks this actually means (eg relative risk reduction).

CLINICAL MANAGEMENT SKILLS

- Consider evaluating his cardiovascular risk and discuss lifestyle changes as an option rather than taking drugs. Be explicit and suggest, if he doesn't mind, that you will talk about the drug later during the consultation (signposting); that way he will feel that you are taking his wishes into account.

- Consider referring him to the smoking cessation clinic if he so wishes.

- Advise on weight management or consider referring him to an obesity clinic (see NICE guidelines on obesity).

- It would be reasonable to check a fasting glucose.

- Check MIMS/BNF on Gold XL in front of him, discussing that the drug hasn't reached the national drug formularies.

- Continue simvastatin for the moment.

- It would be inappropriate to change his drug to Gold XL without being satisfied that it is clinically indicated, safe, superior in effect to simvastatin and cost-effective.

- You are not obliged to prescribe a drug if you don't think that it is appropriate.

- Offer to look at the original research papers on Gold XL and seek advice from the prescribing department at the clinical commissioning group (CCG).

- Once you are more informed about Gold XL, you can drop him a line or invite him in to discuss the matter further. Let him know that you will do this if he wishes.

INTERPERSONAL SKILLS

- What are his ideas on why patients are prescribed statins? Is he concerned that he may be at risk of cardiovascular disease and therefore wants a statin? If so, why? Does he know what the risk factors are for developing heart disease?

- This isn't an easy consultation and it could easily deteriorate to a conflict unless managed carefully.

- Care should be taken not to be patronising or judgemental. Look out for cues; does he appear angry? If so, acknowledge it, or perhaps change the focus of the discussion back to his agenda.

- Offering choices about lifestyle changes is appropriate. Sharing and agreeing a plan that is suitable to both him and you will enhance his satisfaction in your care. He will need support in changing his lifestyle.

- How would he like to be followed up?

- He may not want to engage in a healthy lifestyle, but continue to take statins.

- Would it be reasonable to prescribe a drug as a mandate for him to continue his current lifestyle? It would seem unethical to deny him his current statin if he doesn't want to change his lifestyle.

Note: Gold XL is a fictitious drug in this case.

CHAPTER 6

PREVENTION OF CARDIOVASCULAR DISEASE JOINT BRITISH SOCIETIES' GUIDELINES

TARGET GROUPS	• Established atherosclerotic CVD • Diabetes • Diastolic BP ≥100 mmHg • TC:HDL ≥6.0	• 10 year CVD risk ≥20% • Systolic BP ≥160 mmHg • Elevated BP + target organ damage • Familial dyslipidaemia. Specialist care required.
ASSESSMENT	• Estimate CVD risk using JBS prediction charts (www.bhsoc.org) • Opportunistic risk assessment in over 40s regardless of history – CVD risk <20% repeat within 5 years • CVD risk assessment in younger adults if family history of premature CVD (men <55 years, women <65 years)	

	• Risk assessment should include
	   – Ethnicity
	   – Family CVD history
	   – BP
		– Non-fasting plasma glucose
		– Smoking history
		– Weight and waist circumference
		– Non-fasting lipids or full fasting lipid profile

AIMS	• Reduce BP to <130/80 mmHg in atherosclerotic CVD, diabetes or chronic renal failure • Reduce BP to <140/85 mmHg if asymptomatic and 10-year CVD risk ≥20% • Reduce TC to <4.0 mmol/L or by 25%, whichever is lower • Reduce LDL-C to <2.0 mmol/L or by 30%, whichever is lower • Maintain BMI <25 kg/m² • Maintain waist circumference men <102cm, women <88cm (white Caucasian) • Maintain waist circumference men <90cm, women <80cm (Asian) • Maintain fasting plasma glucose ≤6.0 mmol/L in all high risk patients + HbA1c <6.5% in diabetes	
LIFESTYLE CHANGES	• Lose weight if BMI >25 kg/m² or waist greater than desired limits (see above) • Reduce total fat (≤30% of energy intake); saturated fats (≤10% total fat); increase oily fish consumption • Limit cholesterol to <300 mg per day • 5 portions of fruit and vegetables per day • Limit weekly alcohol to ≤21 units (men); ≤14 units (women) • Reduce salt intake to <6.0 g/day • Take regular exercise, ie 30 mins + aerobic activity per day most days • Stop smoking	

TREATMENT	• Implement statin therapy to achieve TC and LDL-C targets in patients with:
	   – Atherosclerotic CVD
	   – CVD risk ≥20% but asymptomatic
	   – Diabetes ≥40 years
	   – Diabetes 18–39 years + ≥1 of the following: retinopathy; nephropathy; HbA1c >9%; hypertension; TC ≥6 mmol/L; features of metabolic syndrome; family history of premature CVD
	• Implement aspirin 75mg daily (clopidogrel 75mg daily if aspirin not tolerated) in patients with:
	   – Atherosclerotic CVD (once BP controlled)
	   – CVD risk ≥20% but asymptomatic
	   – Diabetes
	• Ensure glycaemic control in diabetes
	• Treat elevated BP
	• Consider anticoagulants in atherosclerotic CVD + high systemic embolism risk
	• Implement beta-blocker therapy following MI
	• Implement ACE inhibitor therapy (or antiotensin II antagonist) in heart failure or left ventricular dysfunction
	   – Also in coronary disease and normal LV function if BP not at target
	   – Also in diabetes with renal dysfunction and microalbuminuria	

Adapted from JBS2: Joint British Societies' guidelines on prevention of cardiovascular disease in clinical practice, 2005.

Fig. 8 Prevention of cardiovascular disease: Joint British Societies' guidelines. Reproduced with the kind permission of MIMS

CHAPTER 6

LIPID MODIFICATION FOR THE PREVENTION OF CARDIOVASCULAR DISEASE NICE GUIDELINE

Adapted from NICE Clinical Guideline 67: Lipid modification – Cardiovascular risk assessment and the modification of blood lipids for the primary and secondary prevention of cardiovascular disease. May 2008; reissued May 2010. www.nice.org.uk

Patients 40 years and over

High-risk groups
- Acute coronary syndrome
- Angina
- Stroke/TIA
- Peripheral vascular disease
- Diabetes (Type I or II)
- Familial lipid disorders
- Over 75 years

SECONDARY PREVENTION

PRIMARY PREVENTION

YES

NO

Acute coronary syndrome
- **Higher intensity statin**
(eg simvastatin 80mg)
- Perform **clinical assessment** and offer **lifestyle advice** (see Box 1).
Note: fasting lipid levels should not be measured until 3 months after starting therapy

Other high-risk groups
- **Simvastatin 40mg***
If potential drug interactions or contraindicated, use lower dose simvastatin or pravastatin
- Perform **clinical assessment** and offer **lifestyle advice** (see Box 1)
Note: management of modifiable risk factors should be performed but must not delay drug treatment

Clinical assessment, lifestyle advice and management of modifiable risk factors
See Box 1
Estimate 10-year CVD risk using Framingham score
See Box 2. CHD risk calculator available at www.mims.co.uk

Targets
TC <4mmol/L (audit level <5mmol/L)
or
LDL-C <2mmol/L

NO

Simvastatin 80mg*
If appropriate

YES

≥20% risk

<20% risk

Simvastatin 40mg*
If potential drug interactions or contraindicated, use lower dose simvastatin or pravastatin

≥20% risk

Risk modifiers
- **Ethnicity**
- **Family history** of premature CHD[†]
- **Other considerations** – low socioeconomic group, BMI >40, antihypertensive or antipsychotic therapy, recently stopped smoking, treated for HIV, connective tissue disease

Ongoing monitoring
- Liver function within 3 months and at 12 months (not again unless clinically indicated)
- Muscle pain, tenderness or weakness
- Peripheral neuropathy (discontinue) and seek specialist advice

<20% risk

Statins not tolerated

- **Review** risk on ongoing basis
- Reinforce **lifestyle advice**

Consider
- Fibrates
- Anion exchange resins/bile acid sequestrants
- Ezetimibe
- Nicotinic acid (secondary prevention only)

KEY:
* or drug of similar efficacy and acquisition cost
† Age at onset <55 years in male relatives and <65 years in female relatives

BOX 1

Clinical Assessment	Lifestyle Advice
BP	Diet and weight
BMI	Physical activity
Fasting blood glucose	Alcohol reduction
Renal function	Smoking cessation
Liver function	
TSH is dyslipidaemia is present	
Smoking status	
Alcohol consumption	
Fasting TC, LDL-C, HDL-C and triglycerides (if not already available)	

BOX 2: RISK ESTIMATION

Risk (including Framingham, ASSIGN and QRISK) equations should not be used for people already considered at high risk of CVD – use clinical assessment instead.

The Framingham equations may overestimate risk in UK populations.

When using these equations, multiply the score by:
- 1.4 for men with a South Asian background
- 1.5 if one relative has a history of premature CHD[†]
- 1.5 to 2.0 if two or more relatives have a history of premature CHD[†]

Framingham CHD risk calculator available at www.mims.co.uk

CHAPTER 6

Fig. 9 Lipid modification for the prevention of cardiovascular disease: NICE guidelines. Reproduced with the kind permission of MIMS

CASE 7

INSTRUCTIONS TO CANDIDATES (CASE NOTES)

You are a locum GP and have never worked in the practice before.

Name	Meredith Jones
Age	19 years
Social and family history	Student
	Asthma review due
Past medical history	Termination of pregnancy, asthma
Best PEFR	420 l/min
Current medication	Microgynon 30
	Salbutamol CFC-free inhaler
	Clenil Modulite 50

BRAINSTORM

INSTRUCTIONS TO ROLE PLAYER (PATIENT)

NOT TO BE SEEN BY CANDIDATE

Patient background:

You are Meredith Jones, aged 19. You are a law student, in Brighton.

You have had a sore throat for 3 days, before which you were well

Opening statement:

'Hiya Doc, I think I need some antibiotics.'

Freely divulged in response to open questions:

You have tried many over-the-counter products.

You feel unwell and are getting worse.

You are able to swallow fluids and food.

The infection hasn't affected your asthma and your cough is dry and non-productive.

Information divulged if asked specifically:

If at all possible, you would like to avoid taking antibiotics as they always give you thrush. You are happy to take a just-in-case prescription in case it gets really bad.

You are allergic to penicillin – it gives you a rash.

You really came to check that it wasn't glandular fever as your best friend died of that after being kicked and his spleen ruptured.

You take your pill regularly and never miss one.

You say that your asthma doesn't bother you.

If asked in more detail, you avoid walking to college but get the bus because you start to wheeze. Come to think of it, you also exercise less because of breathlessness.

Your asthma doesn't affect your sleep.

You don't take your Clenil regularly and you're not sure what it is for.

You don't use your spacer device and are not sure why it is important.

You have a peak flow meter at home, but you're not sure where it is.

You don't smoke.

NOTES

OVERALL AIM OF THE CASE

This case may lead the candidate into assuming that the patient wants antibiotics. The CSA may test the ability of the candidate to perform an asthma review.

DATA-GATHERING, TECHNICAL AND ASSESSMENT SKILLS

- It is important to ascertain whether this patient is unwell, and the examiner may well offer relevant clinical findings.

- She has symptoms of an upper respiratory tract infection (URTI) but it is important to consider whether she has lower respiratory tract symptoms and signs, particularly given that she is asthmatic (auscultate her lungs).

- Severe URTI may present with stridor and/or sepsis. Examination of the throat, assessment for lymphadenopathy and an assessment of systemic involvement should be undertaken – at the very least a temperature and pulse.

- She should be questioned on any drug allergies.

- The latest NICE guidelines on management of URTIs is summarised at the end of this section.

- Her clinical record has an overdue asthma review and you should aim to discuss her asthma, if you have time. If you run out of time, it would be good practice to invite her back to see yourself or the practice nurse for a formal asthma review. Much chronic disease follow-up is performed by practice nurses, many of whom will have training in their chosen fields.

- The May 2008 SIGN/British Thoracic Society guidelines on asthma quote the three Royal College of Physicians' questions on asthma control. In the last week (or month):

CHAPTER 6

- Have your asthma symptoms, including cough, affected your sleep?

- Have you had your usual asthma symptoms during the day (cough/wheeze/SOB/chest tightness)?

- Has your asthma interfered with your usual daily activities?

Tip

✓ **Simply asking: 'How is your asthma doing?' is not acceptable and patients may not realise that they are altering their lifestyle to accommodate their symptoms.**

Asthma reviews in primary care should also include:

- education

- adherence checks

- review of number of exacerbations

- monitoring, eg with spirometry

- inhaler technique

- formulation of personal management plan.

All too often, patients don't understand the role of each inhaler and the benefits of using a spacer device. Patients' understanding should be checked out.

A smoking and occupational history is important with asthma and it's important to ensure they have been offered a full vaccination.

Tip

✓ **Asthma remains a life-threatening condition and it will probably feature in the examination. Note that the SIGN/ BTS asthma guidelines of May 2008, revised in January 2012, are a useful guide.**

CHAPTER 6

CLINICAL MANAGEMENT SKILLS

- Her sore throat should be managed by negotiation. It is important to establish what her expectations are, after all many people don't actually want antibiotics but attend for other reasons.

- If an antibiotic is prescribed, she should be warned about the interaction with the oral contraceptive pill.

- If you think that she may have glandular fever, it would be appropriate to organise a blood test to confirm this and to discuss the risks of splenic rupture in the meantime.

- Education about asthma, its management (including the role of each inhaler), and then formulating a plan tailored to the individual may improve adherence to medication and reduce symptoms.

- Demonstration on inhaler technique may score points if you have time.

- Measuring peak flow will achieve two things in this scenario. First, to demonstrate to the examiner that you know when and how to use a peak flow meter and second, that the patient can use it to regularly monitor the effect of using inhaled corticosteroids (via a spacer device).

- Initiating a peak flow diary is helpful; this may help her manage her asthma more effectively.

INTERPERSONAL SKILLS

- It is important to consider what the patient's concerns are. It is easy to assume that she wants antibiotics. Her concern is whether she has glandular fever.

- If she does have tonsillitis, rather than giving her a prescription for antibiotics, it would be appropriate to give her options, eg over-the-counter medications, a delayed prescription or a definite course of medication.

- Appropriate safety-netting with respect to both asthma and her URTI is required.

- She should be followed up to assess how she is managing with her asthma.

CHAPTER 6

293

KEY POINTS – BTS/SIGN GUIDELINES ON ASTHMA (MAY 2008, REVISED 2012)

DIAGNOSIS (ADULTS)

- \> 1 of wheeze/breathlessness/chest tightness/cough

- Worse at night/with exercise/cold air/allergen exposure

- Atopic history

- Consider with otherwise unexplained low PEFR/FEV_1/eosinophilia (but remember pulmonary eosinophilic syndromes)

- Undertake reversibility testing with spirometry if uncertainty. Use β-agonists or oral steroids, > 400 ml improvement in FEV_1 suggestive of asthma

- Spirometry preferred to peak flow.

MANAGEMENT

- Control defined as:

  - no day/night symptoms

  - no need for rescue medication/no exacerbations

  - no effect on exercise

  - normal lung function

  - minimal drug side effects.

- Primary prevention:

  - encourage mothers to breast-feed

  - avoid tobacco smoke

  - avoid obesity.

- Not enough evidence regarding allergen avoidance, modified milk, vitamins.

- Secondary prevention:
    - reduce house-dust mite
    - allergen-specific immunotherapy
    - control of hyperventilation by using Buteyko breathing – reduces bronchodilator use
    - family therapy.
- Not enough evidence for removing pets/acupuncture/homeopathy/exercise.
- Ionisers have not been shown to be useful.

PHARMACOLOGICAL TREATMENT

- Achieve early control by starting treatment at the appropriate step and then by stepping down to use minimal drugs required to maintain control. This is shown in the stepwise approach to asthma management in adults:

Step 1. Inhaled β agonists.

Step 2. Add in inhaled corticosteroids (ICS).

Step 3. Add in long-acting β agonists (LABAs), stop if no effect, increase dose of ICS if effect not adequate – may require leukotriene antagonists or slow-release theophylline.

Step 4. Increase ICS, add in leukotriene antagonists or slow-release theophylline.

Step 5. Oral steroids; refer.

- Ensure compliance and inhaler technique.
- Patients should use the minimal dose of ICS required.
- Consider 'smart' therapy: patients on step 3 who are not well-controlled may use budesonide/formoterol rather than short-acting β agonist as rescue, as well as a regular preventative inhaler.
- Short-acting β agonists may be taken before exercise.

CHAPTER 6

- Form a management plan with each patient.

- Inhalers and steroids can be used during pregnancy.

KEY POINTS – THE SALMETEROL MULTICENTRE ASTHMA RESEARCH TRIAL (SMART STUDY) 2006

1. Salmetarol vs placebo

2. Randomised control trial (RCT), 26 000 patients

3. Stopped early as increased severe and life-threatening exacerbations with salmetarol especially in African–American individuals.

4. ICS seems to be partially protective against this effect. LABAs should not be used without ICS.

KEY POINTS – NICE GUIDELINES ON RESPIRATORY INFECTIONS, JULY 2008

1. Manage patients' expectations

2. Offer no prescription, delayed prescription or immediate prescription

3. No/delayed prescription considered for:

   - acute otitis media

   - sore throat

   - tonsillitis

   - common cold

   - sinusitis

   - bronchitis

CHAPTER 6

- reassure antibiotics make little immediate difference and have side effects

- safety-net appropriately.

4. Immediate antibiotics may be required depending on clinical presentation in:

- bilateral acute otitis media in children under 2

- acute otitis media with discharge

- acute sore throat with three or more Centor criteria:

  - tonsillar exudate

  - tender/inflamed anterior cervical nodes

  - fever

  - absence of cough

- if systemically very unwell

- if complications, eg pneumonia, quinsy, mastoiditis

- if significant co-morbidities:

  - lung/renal/heart disease, eg heart failure, cystic fibrosis

  - immunosuppressed, ex-premature babies

- > 65 years of age and two of the following or > 80 years of age and one of the following:

  - hospitalised in last year

  - diabetes

  - congestive cardiac failure (CCF)

  - taking steroids.

CASE 8

INSTRUCTIONS TO CANDIDATES (CASE NOTES)

You are a locum GP and have never worked in the practice before.

Name	Lucy Ford
Age	29 years
Social and family history	Social worker
Current Medication	Nil

Last consultation (6 months ago):

URTI

Paracetamol and steam inhalation advised.

Thinking about getting pregnant, discussed.

BRAINSTORM

INSTRUCTIONS TO ROLE PLAYER (PATIENT)
NOT TO BE SEEN BY THE CANDIDATE

Patient background:

You are Lucy Ford, 29 years old and work as a social worker.

You live with your partner and have been trying for a baby for several months.

You are happy and enjoy your job although it can be challenging.

You are very excited as you have missed a period.

Freely divulged in response to open questions

Opening statement:

'I think I may be pregnant doctor, I'm really excited!'

Freely divulged in response to open questions:

Your last period was exactly 7 weeks ago today.

You have been taking folic acid.

You have stopped smoking.

You have done two pregnancy tests which have been positive, but you would like a confirmatory test by the doctor. Your tests were from the local supermarket and you are convinced they are unreliable.

You have never heard of a pregnancy pack/handheld notes.

You have heard the next step is that you meet the midwife to 'book' the pregnancy.

Information divulged if asked specifically:

You don't know that you need to avoid soft cheeses and NSAIDs.

You don't know how much alcohol you can drink; you haven't had a drink for 3 months

You have heard of a special scan to check for Down syndrome but you don't know what it is called. You would want a termination if it was positive.

You have had the rubella vaccination at school.

You have never been pregnant before.

You want to know if you can still go jogging.

You would like to listen to the baby's heartbeat today.

NOTES

OVERALL AIM OF THE CASE

This case requires the candidate to manage a newly pregnant patient.

DATA-GATHERING, TECHNICAL AND ASSESSMENT SKILLS

- Two pregnancy tests are enough to confirm pregnancy. Another is not required, and you should inform her that the tests in the practice are no more sensitive than the commercially available kits.

- When was her last period?

- Is she taking folic acid, does she know why this is important (education is empowering and can increase adherence)?

- Is she avoiding soft cheese? Does she know why she has to (listeria infection)?

- Does she know to avoid NSAIDS and why?

- Is she smoking?

- Does she drink alcohol? She should avoid it if at all possible. *The International Journal of Epidemiology* (Oct 2008) published data suggesting that, at age 3, children of mothers who drank 1–2 units per week did not exhibit behavioural problems or cognitive deficit and in fact boys had less hyperactivity and conduct problems.

- Has she had any abdominal pain or vaginal discharge?

- Check her blood pressure.

- Has she had any terminations or miscarriages?

- Has she a history of disease that may affect the pregnancy? Cardiac, thyroid, diabetes or pelvic injury?

- Has she had a previous ectopic pregnancy?

CHAPTER 6

Tip

> ✓ You cannot always rely on the case summary being complete, as in real life!

CLINICAL MANAGEMENT SKILLS

- Use an obstetric calendar. You can then give her an expected date of delivery.

Tip

> ✓ Remember to bring an obstetric calendar to the CSA and know how to use it!

- Discuss that nuchal scans, in addition to blood tests, provide a risk score for Down syndrome rather than definite yes/no answer.

- She will require a pregnancy pack. (Local practices differ; sometimes doctors give a pack to the woman, and sometimes it is given by the midwife at booking. I suggest that you do as you are used to doing.)

- Discuss the process of booking with the midwife and stress that she will need regular appointments with the midwife and doctor over the course of her pregnancy.

- An easy way to confirm pregnancy in the clinic is to 'listen' for a fetal heart beat with a Doppler ultrasound probe. It is too early to detect a heartbeat at 7 weeks unless a vaginal probe is used. A vaginal probe can detect a heartbeat at 5 weeks and 4 days.

- Jogging shouldn't present any problems.

INTERPERSONAL SKILLS

- As in many cases, summarising what you have said, eg the do's and don'ts of pregnancy, can help her understanding and reinforce your point. You may want to check her understanding by asking explicitly. As in all consultations, ensure that you have understood the patient and the patient has understood you.

- She may or may not take in all of what you say due to the excitement of knowing that she is pregnant. Can you offer her any leaflets, websites or an opportunity to come back if she has questions?

- Women are often full of worry during pregnancy. Ample opportunity should be given for her to express her concerns. Some women may be too shy to ask questions outright but instead offer a cue. Be vigilant for cues and actively listen.

- Explaining the sensitivity of pregnancy tests should be done in language that she understands.

Tip

> ✓ **Suggest that she picks up a leaflet from the waiting room on the way out, or that you'd send her one in the post, rather than promising you'll give it to her at the end of the consultation, unless of course you actually have one! (Emma's diary, a publication from the RCGP, is an excellent manual.)**

KEY POINTS – NICE GUIDELINES ON ANTENATAL CARE, MARCH 2008

1. Woman-centred care.

2. Appropriate access to care.

3. Consider daily 10 mcg vitamin D during pregnancy, and during breast-feeding in at-risk groups, eg south Asians.

CHAPTER 6

4. All pregnant women should be screened for haemoglobinopathies by 10 weeks into pregnancy.

5. Nuchal scan, human chorionic gonadotrophin (hCG) and plasma protein A – for Down syndrome – should be offered from 11^{+0} to 13^{+6} weeks into pregnancy. If women book later, offer a triple/quadruple test at 15–20 weeks.

6. Consider screening for gestational diabetes in high-risk patients, eg high BMI, previous gestational diabetes, family history, previous macrosomic baby, ethnic risk.

7. Those with co-morbidities or previous obstetric complications may require additional care.

8. Advise on alcohol/drugs/smoking.

9. Avoid alcohol for the first 12 weeks of pregnancy if possible.

10. If a woman wants to drink alcohol, the latest NICE guidelines suggest a maximum of 1–2 units/week. Avoid binge drinking.

11. Offer nicotine replacement therapy.

12. Investigate/treat Hb < 11 g/dl.

13. Not routine:

    • breast/pelvic examination

    • weighing

    • screening for chlamydia/streptococcus B (note that screening for group B strep is good practice, see www.gbss.org.uk)

    • fetal movement counting.

CASE 9

INSTRUCTIONS TO CANDIDATES (CASE NOTES)

You are a locum GP and have never worked in the practice before.

Name	Barry Kirk
Age	57 years
Social and family history	Married, two children
Past medical history	Osteoarthritis
	Hypothyroidism
Current medication	Co-codamol 8/500 prn
	Levothyroxine 200 mcg od

Last thyroid function test:

Two years ago; euthyroid. Reminder letter sent to have blood repeated.

BRAINSTORM

INSTRUCTIONS TO ROLE PLAYER (PATIENT)

NOT TO BE SEEN BY THE CANDIDATE

Patient background:

You are Barry Kirk, aged 57, a company director.

You have wear-and-tear arthritis which predominantly affects your knees, probably due to years of rugby.

You take co-codamol intermittently for this.

You've had an under-active thyroid for many years and take levothyroxine daily for this.

Your weight is stable, you are not sensitive to the heat or the cold, and your bowels are normal. Your last thyroid blood test was 2 years ago. You know that you ought to have regular tests and you did receive a letter asking you to have one.

You would like a prostate-specific antigen test (PSA).

Opening statement:

'I'd like a PSA test Doctor!'

Freely divulged in response to open questions:

Your older brother, aged 63, has just been diagnosed with prostate cancer and is scheduled for an operation.

You are worried that you may have prostate cancer.

Your brother saw his GP with a poor urinary stream. His PSA was found to be raised. You don't have any more information than that.

Your urinary stream is strong and you don't dribble urine.

You occasionally have to get up in the night to pass urine.

Information divulged if asked specifically:

You don't have to wait a while before voiding starts.

You have not lost weight.

You don't suffer from erectile dysfunction.

CHAPTER 6

> You don't suffer from any back pain.
>
> As far as you're concerned, a normal PSA excludes prostate and a raised PSA confirms the diagnosis.
>
> You take on board what the doctor says about the PSA test, but would still like it done.
>
> You don't want a rectal examination if asked.

NOTES

OVERALL AIM OF THE CASE

To enable a patient to understand the nuances of the PSA test.

DATA-GATHERING, TECHNICAL AND ASSESSMENT SKILLS

- The primary focus of this case revolves around the patient's fear of having prostate cancer. As such, to gather some information about his brother's case will help you relate this to his own fears and symptoms. For example, his brother had a poor urine flow. You may want to ask if he has that too.

- A full urological history should be taken. In particular, ask about quality of urine flow, frequency, nocturia, haematuria, hesitancy, terminal dribbling and perineal pain. You should also enquire about back and bone pain, weight loss and erectile dysfunction.

- You may want to explain why you are asking about back pain or else he may not understand your questioning, even though you think that you're doing a good job.

- A per rectum examination (PR) would not be allowed in the CSA examination. In any case, disturbing the prostate may elevate the PSA.

- TFTs have not been checked in 2 years. You should enquire about why he hasn't had a blood test; was it the failure of the practice to recall him (assuming that there is a recall system) or did he omit to have the test? In this case, a letter was sent. Did he receive it?

- A cursory review of thyroid symptoms should be taken.

- If appropriate, a brief examination to ensure that he is clinically euthyroid would be appropriate, eg check his pulse rate and rhythm. You would not be expected to perform a formal and full thyroid examination in this situation.

Tip

✓ **Explain to the patient that you are examining him in order to check if he has too much or too little levothyroxine replacement. This will serve to 'sign-post' to the patient what you are doing. Also, it will alert the examiner to what you are doing (like a driving test) and that you are thinking widely.**

CLINICAL MANAGEMENT SKILLS

- Explaining the issues around PSA testing is essential, including the concepts of false-negative and false-positive results, in a way that the patient understands.

- Reiterating the value of annual TFTs should be reinforced. Does he know why this is required?

- Check PSA (if patient would still like this after your discussion) and TFTs. If he had symptoms such as polyuria or nocturia, a blood glucose would also be reasonable. Hypercalcaemia can also cause polyuria.

- Dip-stick the urine for blood, or at least ask for the nurse to do this when he has his blood test (this will save you time during the examination but, more importantly, it is often what we do in daily practice if appropriate).

CHAPTER 6

INTERPERSONAL SKILLS

- The main issue in this case is a discussion about the values of the PSA test. So often patients assume that tests have 100% positive and negative predictive values. To convey this in a way that the patient understands is clearly very important. To score highly, it is worth checking that the patient understands the issues that you have raised regarding PSA.

- Once patients understand that the PSA may be normal in the presence of prostate cancer (up to 20% of cases), and a raised PSA may reflect benign disease but require invasive testing (transrectal biopsy), some may decline the blood test.

- The idea of counselling with respect to the PSA is not necessarily to dissuade patients from having the test, but to inform them of its interpretation.

- This patient is fearful of having cancer. It is important to relieve him of his anxiety or else he will continue to be burdened by fear. He may be reassured by a normal PSA as well as a PR examination. Many patients, despite PSA counselling, will decline a PR examination on the basis of a normal PSA.

- If his PSA is normal, good safety-netting is required. He should be advised to seek advice if he develops lower urinary tact symptoms or haematuria.

- Check that he understands what you mean.

- Appropriate follow-up is required, to discuss the PSA and the thyroid function tests.

FURTHER READING

A good information leaflet about PSA (prostate-specific antigen) testing for prostate cancer can be found at: www.cancerscreening.nhs.uk/prostate/prostate-patient-info-sheet.pdf

CHAPTER 6

CASE 10

INSTRUCTIONS TO CANDIDATES (CASE NOTES)

You are a locum GP and have never worked in the practice before.

Name	Sarah Reynolds
Age	39 years
Social and family history	Non-smoker
Past medical history	Coeliac disease
Current medication	Nil

BRAINSTORM

INSTRUCTIONS TO ROLE PLAYER (PATIENT)

NOT TO BE SEEN BY THE CANDIDATE

Patient background:

You are Sarah Reynolds, a marketing executive.

You're 39, about to have your 40th birthday.

You live on your own and have a very high-powered job.

You have had coeliac disease for 20 years and are meticulous about your diet.

You are regularly followed up by your private gastroenterologist and have no complications related to coeliac disease. You don't want to discuss coeliac disease today.

Opening statement:

'I've been getting headaches, Doctor.'

Freely divulged in response to open questions:

Your headaches have been occurring for 3 months and are getting worse.

They feel like a tight band around your forehead.

The headaches occur almost every day.

They seemed to go while you were away on holiday.

Information divulged if asked specifically:

You don't have a cold.

You haven't been involved in any trauma.

They don't wake you up, but you often find you have them in the mornings.

You don't vomit with them but sometimes feel quite sick.

They do not occur in clusters (clusters = every day for a few days followed by weeks or months without a headache).

You don't suffer any visual disturbance, aura or neurological disturbance.

You don't have any neck stiffness.

You haven't had your eyes tested in 2 years.

You think that you have migraines.

You don't smoke but drink three gin and tonics (1 unit each) to relax at night.

Your last period was 3 weeks ago. They are regular.

You're not sexually active; work is so busy and stressful that you don't have time for a relationship. This is upsetting because you're nearly 40 and are desperate to have children. You feel that your biological clock is ticking.

You are happy in yourself but work is very stressful. It involves a lot of deadlines and millions of pounds rest on your shoulders.

You find it difficult getting off to sleep, and wake early thinking about work.

You have used your mother's codeine tablets daily to help with the headaches.

NOTES

OVERALL AIM OF THE CASE

The aim of this case is to test the candidate's ability to distinguish between sinister and benign causes of headaches while consulting in a patient-centred way.

DATA-GATHERING, TECHNICAL AND ASSESSMENT SKILLS

- The differential diagnosis of headache is vast. In this case the patient has stress headaches.

- The diagnosis is usually made from careful history taking.

- Exclusion of sinister and important conditions is imperative.

- The aetiology of a chronic headache should be borne in mind during the consultation: tension, medication overuse, chronic sinusitis, eye strain/disease, carbon monoxide poisoning, migraine, cluster headaches, raised intracranial pressure (eg neoplastic disease).

- Examination includes blood pressure, fundscopy, visual fields, head and neck. Examination in her case is normal.

- Her blood pressure should be checked.

- It is important to ensure that she isn't depressed, perhaps by appropriate questioning of biological and cognitive features of depression or by asking her to fill in a validated questionnaire.

- While a short review of her coeliac disease would be appropriate, she is not keen in this case.

Tip

✓ **If this patient were older, temporal arteritis would need to be excluded.**

CLINICAL MANAGEMENT SKILLS

- This patient is likely to have tension headaches secondary to her stressful job. The headaches may also be related to regular analgesia use or eye strain, particularly if she has a busy job and spends hours in front of a computer screen.

- She should be advised to see her optician for an eye check and to refrain from using regular analgesia.

CHAPTER 6

- Her stress should be managed in a way that is suitable to both you and herself. Options include changing her work pattern and counselling.

- Exercise is frequently therapeutic.

- Alcohol can cause headaches; her intake should be discussed.

- You may elect to check her FBC and calcium. Hypercalcaemia and polycythaemia can cause headache.

INTERPERSONAL SKILLS

- It is crucial to reassure the patient and help her see what the causes of her headaches are likely to be. Many patients with headaches fear a tumour. Her fears should be explored, without assuming what her particular concerns actually are. It would be a catastrophe to make her worried about a condition that she hadn't considered. In this case she is concerned about migraine rather than a brain tumour. Migraine should be discussed to put her fears at rest.

- She must feel enabled to choose a management plan that she is comfortable with. By giving her treatment options, she can decide what treatment she prefers.

- Follow-up is essential to check if the headaches have settled and to offer support.

KEY POINTS AND FURTHER READING

1. Migraine

   - periodic headache

   - 80% of patients experience their first migraine before the age 30

   - classic: prodrome, eg mood/appetite change followed by visual/ sensory aura

CHAPTER 6

- common: no aura
- followed by throbbing unilateral headache, nausea, photophobia, phonophobia
- lasts 4–72 hours
- may have unilateral lacrimation
- reversible neurological signs, eg hemiplegia
- may result in stroke (rare)
- patient should not have the oral contraceptive pill if she is at risk of stroke, migraine lasts > 72 hours, focal aura or if she needs ergotamine
- treatment: over-the-counter medication, antiemetics, $5HT_1$ – receptor agonists and ergotamine.

2. Cluster headaches
   - males > females
   - onset 25–50 years
   - clusters last days to weeks; headaches occur daily during this period
   - remissions last months
   - unilateral severe headache – lasts up to an hour at a time
   - lacrimation and ipsilateral red eye
   - may cause: Horner syndrome, retro-orbital pain, nasal congestion
   - treatment: oxygen, $5HT_1$ - receptor agonists and ergotamine
   - steroids may be used
   - verapamil may be used as prophylaxis.
   - SIGN (Scottish Intercollegiate Guidelines Network). Diagnosis and management of headache in adults. Edinburgh: SIGN, 2008. www.sign.ac.uk

CHAPTER 6

CASE 11

INSTRUCTIONS TO CANDIDATES (CASE NOTES)

You are a locum GP and have never worked in the practice before.

Name	Nora Howell
Age	73 years
Social and family history	Lives by herself
Past medical history	Polymyalgia rheumatica, 12 months
	Osteoarthritis
	Anxiety
	Hypertension
	Basal cell carcinoma, 2004
Current medication	Prednisolone 8 mg od
	Paracetamol 1g qds
	Lercanidipine 10 mg od
Blood pressure (last week):	138/81 mmHg
Fasting blood sugar (last week):	5.8 mmol/l

Previous consultation:

Malignancy excluded

Normal U&Es

Wedge fracture seen on spinal radiograph (T4)

Plan DEXA scan and review

DEXA scan (2 weeks ago): spinal T score: -2.9

Hip T score: -3.2

Suggest vitamin D/calcium and bisphosphonates

BRAINSTORM

Tip

> ✓ If you don't know what the medications are for in the case notes, use your BNF before the patient comes into the room.

INSTRUCTIONS TO ROLE PLAYER (PATIENT)

NOT TO BE SEEN BY THE CANDIDATE

Patient background:

You are Nora Howell, you are 73 years old.

You are a retired dinner lady and live on your own.

Your two children live about 100 miles away.

You have come to get the results of your osteoporosis (DEXA) scan which you had 2 weeks ago.

Opening statement:

'Hello Doctor, we've not met before! I've come to get the results of my scan.'

Freely divulged in response to open questions:

You've been on prednisolone for a year for polymyalgia rheumatica.

You have had severe back pain for the last 2 months. Your GP organised a lot of blood tests which were normal. An X-ray showed a damaged bone in the back. A scan was organised to look at your bones but you're not exactly sure what it was looking for.

You are currently taking prednisolone (8 mg) every day, although you occasionally forget to take them.

You don't have any muscle stiffness around your neck and shoulders and feel the steroids work well.

Information divulged if asked specifically:

You have not had any weight loss or night sweats.

Your friend has been prescribed prednisolone for a skin disease and she is also taking tablets to help her bones, although you don't know what the tablets do to bones. You are cross that you weren't given bone tablets.

You are worried about the bone scan; you were told by one of your friends that this was to look for cancer that has spread to the bones, particularly as you had a skin cancer a few years ago.

You have never smoked or drunk alcohol. You have never fallen and are steady on your feet.

NOTES

OVERALL AIM OF THE CASE

This case asks the candidate to deliver an abnormal result and manage an angry patient.

DATA-GATHERING, TECHNICAL AND ASSESSMENT SKILLS

- The scan results indicate osteoporosis.

- It is likely the patient's osteoporosis has been caused by prednisolone.

- Bisphosphonates ought to have been considered when she was initiated on steroids.

- Other causes of osteoporosis may be considered if relevant:

  - posmenopausal, age-related, multiparity, family history, alcohol, smoking, Cushing's disease, hyperparathyroidism, prolactinoma, hyperthyroidism, ciclosporin, myeloma, ulcerative colitis, renal failure, Turner syndrome.

  - DXA scans compare the patient's bone density to the population mean peak density (eg young adults of same sex).

CHAPTER 6

- It is expressed as standard deviations (SD) from the mean.

• T score down to	–1	normal
• T score	–1 to –2.5	oesteopenia
• T score below	–2.5	osteoporosis

  - Fracture risk increases twofold with every SD.
  - Fracture risk increases by 1.5/every 10 years of life over the age of 30.

- Important features to cover include steroid compliance and ensuring that she knows never to stop them suddenly. Does she know why?

- She should be assessed for her risk of falls.

- How is the condition affecting her quality of life?

- Examination of the shoulder girdle and ensuring that she doesn't have symptoms of temporal arteritis is appropriate.

CLINICAL MANAGEMENT SKILLS

- Given that she has significant osteoporosis with evidence of wedge fracture, calcium and vitamin D supplements in addition to bisphosphonates should be prescribed. The regimen (eg weekly alendronate sodium, taken before breakfast while remaining upright) should be explained. Explain the side effects of weekly bisphosphonates and check that she is still willing to take them.

- A steroid card should be issued (for the purposes of the examination, you may elect to send one in the post), and it would be prudent to check her understanding of the side effects of steroids.

- An erythrocyte sedimentation rate (ESR) should be organised for polymyalgia rheumatica (PMR) disease monitoring. Her blood pressure and blood glucose should also be monitored regularly.

- If her polymyalgia is quiescent, the prednisolone dose should be reduced to 7 mg od.

- A discussion about pain control (for spinal pain) should take place.

INTERPERSONAL SKILLS

- This patient, perhaps rightly so, is upset that she wasn't given bisphosphonates when she was first commenced on steroids. It would be reasonable to acknowledge her feelings and explore with her what, if anything, she'd like you to do. You may offer to investigate the notes, and it would be good clinical governance to hold a significant event analysis. She may want to hear the outcome of the analysis. This approach is more appropriate than a defensive one.

- She may not fully understand what osteoporosis is. Patients often become confused between osteoarthritis, -porosis and -malacia. Checking out her knowledge of osteoporosis will score highly.

- What are her concerns? In this case, cancer? Can you explain why this isn't cancer, in language that she understands and using her own health beliefs? You may start by asking her why she thinks that she may have cancer affecting her bones. What is her knowledge of basal cell cancer and its potential for spread?

- Explaining what she may expect from osteoporosis drugs is important. Does she expect them to cure her pain? Does she know how long she has to take the drugs for?

- Discuss her options so that management can be shared and she feels empowered.

- It is crucial that you summarise the discussion that you have with her and check that she understands the issues that have been raised.

- She should be followed up to assess how she is getting on with her medication, and a follow-up DXA scan may be arranged in the longer term to assess the change in *T* score.

FURTHER READING

The National Osteoporosis Guideline Group (NOGG) www.shef.ac.uk/NOGG

The FRAX® fracture risk assessment tool www.shef.ac.uk/FRAX

CHAPTER 6

CASE 12

INSTRUCTIONS TO CANDIDATES (CASE NOTES)

You are a locum GP and have never worked in the practice before.

Name   Unknown

The computers have crashed and you have no access to her notes. You have never met this patient before.

BRAINSTORM

INSTRUCTIONS TO ROLE PLAYER (PATIENT)

NOT TO BE SEEN BY THE CANDIDATE

Patient background:

You are Holly Gibbs, aged 22. You are unemployed.

You are very defensive because you are often treated like a drug addict.

You would like a month's supply of diazepam, which you pronounce diazepa<u>n</u>.

Opening statement:

'I'd like some more diazepam.'

Freely divulged in response to open questions:

You have two children, one of 6 years and another of 3 years.

You don't have any other medical problems

You are not allergic to any medicines. You live in a rough part of town.

You've started an A-level course to make a better life for you and your children.

You don't have time for friends and you find it difficult to trust anyone.

Information divulged if asked specifically:

You hate living there; it has a reputation for drug and social problems and you worry about its effect on your children.

You were fostered from the age of nine, following the death of your parents.

You take diazepam, 5 mg three times a day, for anxiety since being raped 4 years ago.

You get the shakes if you don't take them.

You never take more than you're supposed to and would love to come off them. You have never sold diazepam to anyone else.

You don't pay for prescriptions.

You saw a psychiatrist and a rape counsellor on a fortnightly basis for a year regarding the rape.

You haven't been sleeping and your appetite and weight have dropped over the last 2 months

You feel that your concentration is non-existent and that you can't remember a thing.

You haven't enjoyed life for the last 3 months.

Life is worth living, only for the sake of your children, otherwise you'd end it.

You would never harm your children.

You don't hear voices and have no paranoid symptoms.

You have never taken illicit drugs.

You don't drink alcohol or smoke.

You are concerned that you may be depressed.

You'd rather not have any more tablets, but you found the counselling helpful and are keen to have more sessions.

NOTES

DATA-GATHERING, TECHNICAL AND ASSESSMENT SKILLS

We realise how reliant we are on technology when it fails.

- Establish her history; how much diazepam does she take, what dose and why she takes it?

- What is her current mental status?

- Is she depressed or anxious? Ask about features of depression and anxiety.

- Consider using a validated questionnaire to quantify the extent of her depression and anxiety.

- Are there features of bipolar disorder?

- Is she suicidal?

- Is she functioning on a day-to-day basis?

- What is her social status?

- Does she take illicit drugs?

- Who is her usual doctor?

- Is she coping with the children?

- What are her views on diazepam use?

Tip

✓ **The Royal College of General Practitioners offers a course in managing drug misuse, while NICE have published information on addiction, including opiate detoxification and psychological interventions.**

CLINICAL MANAGEMENT SKILLS

- As you don't know her, you may be uncomfortable in prescribing a month's supply of diazepam. It would be reasonable, however, to prescribe a small amount and follow her up regularly until you gain each other's trust.

- Consider weaning her off diazepam, if she is ready to. How would you do that?

- Frequent follow-up, if she agrees, would provide a supportive environment for her.

- Organise counselling or antidepressants, or both, depending on what she wants.

CHAPTER 6

INTERPERSONAL SKILLS

- It is very easy to assume that this patient is a drug addict in need of diazepam.

- Apologise for having to take the full history again. Explaining that the computers have crashed will go a long way to making her feel at ease, establishing trust and making her less defensive.

- Sensitivity to her history is crucial to grain trust.

- What are her concerns? She may be worried about coming off diazepam; in particular she may worry about becoming more anxious, and whether she will ever get better.

- What are her expectations? How will she come off the diazepam? What will happen if she starts to withdraw? What will a counsellor do? Is she concerned that antidepressants are addictive?

- Share management by offering options, eg counselling or antidepressants, which will empower her to take control of her health.

- She will need frequent follow-up and support.

CHAPTER 6

CASE 13

INSTRUCTIONS TO CANDIDATES (CASE NOTES)

You are a locum GP and have never worked in the practice before.

Name	Joseph Stotter
Age	79 years
Social and family history	Lives with son and his family
	Wife died 12 years ago
	Retired plumber
Past medical history	Atrial fibrillation
	Transient ischaemic attack
	Hypertension
	COPD
	Osteoarthritis
	Umbilical hernia repair
	Appendicectomy
	Femoral fracture (road traffic accident, 1978)
Current medication	Warfarin 3 mg od
	Simvastatin 40 mg nocte
	Ramipril 5 mg od
	Amlodipine 5 mg od
	Bisoprolol 1.25 mg od
	Salbutamol CFC free inhaler
	Tiotropium inhaler 18 mg od
	Paracetamol 500 mg 2 qds
	Tramadol 50 mg 2 qds

Mr Stotter saw Dr Rose last week complaining of upper back pain. He arranged some blood and urine tests:

Hb 10.9 g/dl

ESR 99 mm/h

PSA 0.5 ng/ml

Calcium: normal

Protein electrophoresis: monoclonal band

Urine: positive for Bence Jones protein

BRAINSTORM

Tip

✓ The case notes may appear complicated but read through them carefully; it may be, as in this case, that the majority of the information is background rather than directly relevant to today's consultation.

INSTRUCTIONS TO ROLE PLAYER (PATIENT)

NOT TO BE SEEN BY THE CANDIDATE

Patient background:

You are Joseph Stotter, age 79

You've come to get your blood test results; the doctor insisted last week that you come in to get the blood results.

Opening statement:

'Hello Doctor, I've come to get my results.'

Freely divulged in response to open questions:

You have been suffering upper back pain for a few months.

The pain has been getting worse and for 2 weeks has been waking you up at night time.

You don't have night sweats but you have lost some weight.

You have not suffered any trauma to your back.

Information divulged if asked specifically:

You have had a cough for years, due to your COPD.

You have never coughed up any blood.

Your bowels are normal.

The pain is so bad that paracetamol and tramadol are not controlling the pain.

You have tried physiotherapy and seen a chiropractor with no improvement.

Your urine flow has been normal.

You want a scan for osteoporosis.

Your wife had osteoporosis and you are convinced that is what you have.

You have no idea what the blood tests were for; you think they were for osteoporosis.

You have started smoking again but you never smoke near the grandchildren and only smoke outside.

You never drink alcohol.

NOTES

DATA-GATHERING, TECHNICAL AND ASSESSMENT SKILLS

- This patient has come to the get the results of his blood tests.

- While it is important to review his history, the focus of the consultation is to manage a new diagnosis of myeloma.

- Given he has back pain, how severe is it? What medications is he taking? Does he get side effects? Does he have leg weakness or experience difficulty in passing urine?

CLINICAL MANAGEMENT SKILLS

- This patient has anaemia, a monoclonal band on protein electrophoresis and Bence Jones proteins in his urine (note: in around 20% of cases, patients will have Bence Jones proteins without a monoclonal band. It is therefore imperative that urine is sent for Bence Jones protein if myeloma is suspected).

CHAPTER 6

- It would seem reasonable to re-check his Hb to see if there is a downward trend, and to re-check calcium (often raised in myeloma) and renal function ('myeloma kidney').

- Analgesia should be discussed.

- A 2WW referral should be made to the haematology department.

INTERPERSONAL SKILLS

- As with every patient, welcome the patient, make him feel at ease.

- Asking the patient the story so far may put him at ease and give him the opportunity to express his concerns (eg osteoporosis). It will also provide an ideal starting point to the consultation. Check his understanding: does he actually know what osteoporosis is?

- Does he look concerned? Does he offer a cue? 'You look worried … is there something on your mind …?'

- Part of the consultation is about breaking bad news. It may be more appropriate for you to explain that you think there is 'something worrying … something more sinister than osteoporosis … a lesion in your back' and see what his reaction is.

- You may want to involve his health beliefs: 'The tests show something more serious than osteoporosis.'

- Check his understanding: does he understand your concern that he has a potentially serious illness?

- You may need to be more explicit, but be sensitive: 'The hospital will need to confirm it, but I think that you may have a type of cancer in your back.'

- Offer hope: 'The diagnosis still needs to be confirmed … there are treatments available.'

- Sensitivity is important.

- The use of silence is useful.

CHAPTER 6

- Does he have concerns? Will he die? What will the treatment be? Will his pain get worse? How long has he got? This consultation can easily run over 10 minutes: time management is important. It would be worth explaining that the diagnosis has to be confirmed first and these are questions that the specialist is better placed to answer.

- Would he like to come back soon, perhaps with a family member and for a longer appointment, to discuss the matter further?

- Is he agreeable to an urgent referral?

- What are his expectations? Does he know/want to know what the hospital process is? He may need a marrow biopsy.

- He should contact the surgery if he doesn't hear from the hospital within the week.

- Confirm his contact details so that the hospital sends the appointment to the right address.

FURTHER READING

NICE have published a very practical guide to metastatic spine disorders, essential reading for the CSA.

NICE. *Metastatic spinal cord compression: diagnosis and management of adults at risk of and with metastatic spinal cord compression.* London: NICE, 2008. www.nice.org.uk/guidance/CG75.

BONUS CASE

IN THIS STATION ...

You are a duty GP in the practice.

MATERIALS AND INSTRUCTIONS TO CANDIDATE (CASE NOTES)

Name	Holly Brown
Age	56 years
Address	90 Bedford Close, London W1
Social and family history	Lives on own
	Artist
Past medical history	Nil
Current medication	Nil

BRAINSTORM

EXAMINATION FINDINGS
Information offered on iPad if appropriate

Right facial drooping

Forehead also affected

Right eyelid able to protect eye

No vesicles in right ear

No parotid masses

No glands in neck

No other neurological abnormalities

No cardiovascular abnormalities

CHAPTER 6

INSTRUCTIONS TO ROLE PLAYER (PATIENT)

NOT TO BE SEEN BY THE CANDIDATE

You are Holly Brown, an artist.

You developed drooping of the right side of your face overnight.

You feel fine in yourself.

You're worried that you've had a stroke.

You're very worried about taking steroids (if offered) but reluctantly take them.

Opening statement

'Hello doctor, help me, I'm having a stroke!'

Freely divulged in response to open questions:

You were fine last night.

You woke feeling fine in the morning but were horrified to see the right side of your face drooping when you looked in the mirror.

Information divulged if asked specifically:

You are not experiencing any headache/visual disturbance/pain/limb weakness/speech difficulties

You're concerned that you're having a stroke.

You've dribbled a little from the corner of your mouth.

You're able to fully close your eyes.

You've never heard of Bell's palsy.

Your concerns about steroids are related to putting on weight and becoming hairy. You didn't realise that steroids can cause other complications. Nevertheless, you're happy to take them.

You've never heard of the 111 service.

NOTES

OVERALL AIM OF THE CASE

The aim of the case is to confidentially diagnose Bell's palsy, exclude other causes of a nerve VII palsy and manage it appropriately.

DATA GATHERING, TECHNICAL AND ASSESSMENT SKILLS

- The key issues here are to identify that this patient has a lower motor neuron palsy.

- Recognition that the forehead is also affected is the main clinical give-away in distinguishing a lower from an upper motor neuron disorder.

- The next logical step is to establish the cause, eg Bell's palsy, Ramsay Hunt syndrome, parotid tumour, trauma and so on.

- Zoster vesicles in the ipsilateral ear suggest Ramsay Hunt syndrome

CLINICAL MANAGEMENT SKILLS

- High-dose steroids (60–80 mg prednisolone) for 5 days, followed by a 10-day taper should be offered.

- Consider aciclovir.

- Safety netting, eg does she know about the new 111 service?

- Appropriate and regular follow-up.

INTERPERSONAL SKILLS

- Recognise that this is a frightening experience for the patient.

- Ensure that the patient feels confident in what you're saying and that she has a clear understanding of the situation at hand.

CHAPTER 6

- Ensure understanding of what to do practically if concerned.
- Offer reassurance and hope.

KEY POINTS (BELL'S PALSY)

- Most facial palsies are Bell's palsies
- Rapid onset
- Lower motor neuron (hence no forehead sparing)
- Dribbling, eating and difficulties closing the ipsilateral eye can occur
- Corneal ulceration can occur if the patient cannot adequately blink. in which case lubrication, a patch or even tarsorrhaphy.

CHAPTER 6

Chapter 7
Exam Circuit 4

Case Number	1	2	3	4	5	6	7	8	9	10	11	12	13
The general practice consultation	✓	✓	✓	✓	✓	✓	✓	✓	✓	✓	✓	✓	✓
Clinical governance							✓						
Patient safety				✓	✓	✓		✓		✓			
Clinical ethics and values-based practice	✓	✓		✓		✓	✓						
Promoting equality and valuing diversity													
Evidence-based practice												✓	
Research and academic activity													
Teaching, mentoring and clinical supervision													
Management in primary care					✓	✓							
Information management and technology													
Healthy people: promoting health and preventing disease									✓		✓		
Genetics in primary care													
Care of acutely ill people				✓						✓			
Care of children and young people									✓				
Care of older adults					✓					✓	✓		
Women's health		✓				✓		✓					
Men's health							✓						
Sexual health						✓	✓						
Care of people with cancer and palliative care											✓		
Care of people with mental health problems								✓					
Care of people with learning disabilities													
Cardiovascular problems													✓
Digestive problems					✓					✓			
Drug and alcohol problems													
ENT and facial problems				✓									
Eye problems													
Metabolic problems												✓	
Neurological problems													
Respiratory problems				✓									
Rheumatology and conditions of the musculoskeletal system (including trauma)	✓		✓										
Skin problems											✓		

Fig. 10 Circuit 4 cases plotted against RCGP curriculum

CHAPTER 7

CASE 1

INSTRUCTIONS TO CANDIDATES (CASE NOTES)

You are a locum doctor, you have never met this patient before.

Name	Robin Greeves
Age	39 years
Social and family history	Postman, married, two children
Past medical history	Recurrent mechanical back pain
	MRI (back) 3 months ago: normal
Current medication	Ibuprofen

BRAINSTORM

INSTRUCTIONS TO ROLE PLAYER (PATIENT)

NOT TO BE SEEN BY THE CANDIDATE

Patient background:

You are Robin Greeves. You are 39 years old and you work as a postman.

You have suffered from recurrent back pain for the last 8 years since falling off a chair.

You have seen a specialist and been thoroughly investigated, including blood tests and a recent MRI scan.

Opening statement:

'I need a doctor's certificate.'

Freely divulged in response to open questions:

You have come to get another medical certificate.

You want the certificate to cover you for last week, backdated to 7 days ago.

Information divulged if asked specifically:

You have taken many days off work over the years.

Your manager is unhappy about the number of days that you have taken off in the past.

You last saw a doctor 3 months ago, for a certificate.

Your pain is better now.

It was the same pain as you always get.

You have no problems passing urine, no numbness or pins and needles.

If you don't get a doctor's certificate, you run the risk of being disciplined or even sacked.

You couldn't come in last week to get a certificate because you were in too much pain and you didn't want to bother the doctor for a home visit. You took paracetamol for the pain.

NOTES

DATA-GATHERING, TECHNICAL AND ASSESSMENT SKILLS

- The patient hasn't come to discuss back pain but to get a medical certificate.

- A medical certificate may be given had he seen a doctor in the last month, and if the notes warrant a certificate.

- How does he manage his pain?

- Ask why he didn't seek advice when he was in pain – that's what most people do.

- Is he aware of the rules surrounding medical certification? Does he know about the rules on self-certification?

- Is he aware that doctors may be investigated if they issue certificates fraudulently?

CLINICAL MANAGEMENT SKILLS

- A medical certificate cannot be given on the basis of a patient's own say so.

- A Med 3 certificate cannot be given retrospectively. Many patients don't appreciate this.

- He may be given a private letter stating that he was unwell with back pain the previous week. GPs may charge for this.

INTERPERSONAL SKILLS

• This can be a challenging consultation: testing a doctor's probity and knowledge of medical certification.

• It would be easy to give the patient a certificate but that would not be in keeping with the rules stated in the obligations for doctors to issue certificates.

• Knowingly issuing a certificate would be inappropriate irrespective of the consequences for the patient. Telling him you are obliged to operate by the rules, and that not doing so may lead to sanctions being brought against you, is likely to pacify him.

• It may be helpful to educate the patient on rules surrounding medical certificates.

• Offering the option of a private letter stating the patient's story may be acceptable to him.

• If he gets aggressive, when a certificate is not given, it is worth acknowledging how frustrating it must be for him.

• However guilty he makes you feel, you should not break the rules set out in the law.

CHAPTER 7

CASE 2

INSTRUCTIONS TO CANDIDATES (CASE NOTES)

Name	Annette Johnson
Age	35 years
Social and family history	Single, solicitor
Past medical history	Ovarian cancer, curative surgery 4 weeks ago

BRAINSTORM

INSTRUCTIONS TO ROLE PLAYER (PATIENT)

NOT TO BE SEEN BY THE CANDIDATE

Patient background:

You are Annette Johnson, you are 35 years old. You live alone and have a very busy job as a solicitor.

You appear anxious.

You have come to the doctor to express your gratitude for diagnosing your ovarian cancer. The doctor's prompt action meant that you could have curative surgery.

You are so thankful for the care that you received.

You have heard of many legal cases where the doctor has failed to diagnose the cancer and you understand that it is a notoriously difficult cancer to diagnose early.

You have made a full recovery and have been back at work for a week.

Things are going well at work and you are very happy there. Your boss is being very supportive.

Opening statement:

'I'd like to give you something.'

Freely divulged in response to open questions:

You would like to express your gratitude by giving the doctor a watch – the watch is worth £1000.

You won't take no for an answer.

You feel that you owe your life to your doctor.

You are seeing your oncologist next week.

Information divulged if asked specifically:

You understand that it is against the General Medical Council (GMC) guidelines but you won't say anything to them.

You are scared that the cancer may return.

You have recurrent nightmares about dying and being in pain.

You also have nightmares about never having children, although you have been told that you should be able to conceive with help.

You don't feel depressed.

You are eating well.

You sometimes get panic attacks, they come out of the blue, last a few minutes and you feel breathless as if you are going to die.

NOTES

DATA-GATHERING, TECHNICAL AND ASSESSMENT SKILLS

- Little knowledge about ovarian cancer is required in this case.

Tip

   ✓ **Always admit the limits of your knowledge to the patient rather than trying to hash together a half-right solution to her needs.**

- It would be good practice to ask how she is doing and assess if she has come to terms with her condition. Has she recovered from the treatment?

- Panic attacks are commonplace; it is not surprising that she is suffering from them. What brings them on?

- Anxiety and depression often coincide; screening for depression would be appropriate.

- Quantifying how severe her depression and anxiety are by a validated questionnaire is appropriate.

CLINICAL MANAGEMENT SKILLS

- You may want to offer her counselling or SSRIs for her panic attacks.

- Self-help books and websites such as Moodgym (http://moodgym. anu.edu.au/welcome) are invaluable and empowering.

INTERPERSONAL SKILLS

- She should be followed up appropriately regarding her panic attacks.

- Exploring her ideas about how and why people (and herself) get panic attacks may be therapeutic.

- Many patients fear being prescribed psychiatric drugs. Often, when given the choice, patients prefer non-pharmacological management. Sharing management options will empower her.

- Accepting an expensive gift can adversely affect the doctor–patient relationship and may be considered a conflict of interest. There have been a number of GMC cases surrounding this subject. The Social Care Bill (2000) legislated that gifts over £100 in value should be declared.

- A gift may alter the dynamic between the doctor and patient such that the patient may expect preferential treatment and the doctor feels beholden.

- Explaining to the patient that receiving such gifts would not be in keeping with guidance set out by the GMC would be appropriate. While she may insist that you take the watch, it would be advisable to stick with the GMC guidance in a way that won't cause offence and maintain your professional integrity.

KEY POINTS AND FURTHER READING

The GMC offers robust guidance that must be followed and states:

'You must not ask for or accept any inducement, gift or hospitality which may affect or be seen to affect the way you prescribe for, treat or refer patients. You must not offer such inducements to colleagues.'

CASE 3

INSTRUCTIONS TO CANDIDATES (CASE NOTES)

You are a locum in a busy general practice. One of the partners in the practice has a very good reputation in managing musculoskeletal disorders.

Name	Henry Carter
Age	39 years
Social and family history	CEO, Carter Computers International
Past medical history	Recurrent ear infections
	Ankle sprain
	Stress at work
	Tibial fracture (road traffic accident 1992)

Examination findings

Left shoulder is painful, with reduced range of movement especially upon external rotation and abduction. Pain is elicited on active and passive shoulder movements.

BRAINSTORM

INSTRUCTIONS TO ROLE PLAYER (PATIENT)

NOT TO BE SEEN BY THE CANDIDATE

Patient background:

You are 39-year-old Henry Carter, the owner of a successful computer company.

You have had left shoulder pain for the past 4 months.

You are right handed.

The shoulder also feels stiff and you can't move it as much you normally can; even reaching to your back pocket is difficult.

Opening statement:

'I'd like to see a specialist.'

Freely divulged in response to open questions:

It is affecting your sleep, waking you when you turn. You can't lie on your left side.

You would like a referral to an orthopaedic consultant. You don't have private insurance as you believe in the NHS, although you think the Labour Government has destroyed it.

Information divulged if asked specifically:

It is starting to affect your quality of life.

Your performance at work is suffering.

You are getting short tempered and your girlfriend made you come to the doctor.

You have recently started going to the gym and think your pain may be related to weight training, although you haven't been able to train recently, because of the pain.

You have heard of a frozen shoulder, but you are not quite sure what it is.

CHAPTER 7

NOTES

DATA-GATHERING, TECHNICAL AND ASSESSMENT SKILLS

- This patient describes an adhesive capsulitis of the shoulder.
- It is relevant to explore how the pain came about and the effect on his quality of life.
- The assessment should include an examination of the shoulder in order to exclude other pathologies and to confirm the diagnosis.
- It is important to inspect the shoulder to ensure that there are no scars or swellings. Is there any muscle wasting?
- Is there any evidence of tenderness, crepitus or effusion within the joint and supporting structures?
- Check the patient's range of movements, active and passive. He should be seated comfortably.
- Assess the joints, rotator cuff and for a frozen shoulder.
- The diagnosis of adhesive capsulitis is a clinical one.

CLINICAL MANAGEMENT SKILLS (ADHESIVE CAPSULITIS)

- Analgesia, paracetamol, NSAIDs
- TENS machine
- Physiotherapy if combined with intra-articular injection of steroid
- Patient education
- Side effects of NSAIDs should be discussed.

INTERPERSONAL SKILLS

- This patient would like to see an orthopaedic surgeon. What does he hope to gain from this?

- Establishing what the patient knows about 'frozen shoulder' and educating him on its pathology and treatment are empowering. Based on this new knowledge, he may change his view about wanting a referral to an orthopaedic surgeon. Offer leaflets to reinforce what you have said.

- What are his expectations? Symptoms may persist for up to 3 years.

- Offering management options before a surgical referral will again empower the patient and make him feel involved in his own care.

- Inviting the patient to see your colleague (which can be organised quickly) who has a special interest in musculoskeletal diseases and who is used to managing his condition is entirely appropriate.

- If he is still keen to see an orthopaedic surgeon, it may be worth indicating that the surgeon may also try an injection, but it may take several weeks before he is seen.

CHAPTER 7

CASE 4: TELEPHONE CONSULTATION

INSTRUCTIONS TO CANDIDATES (CASE NOTES)

Name	Thomas Protheroe
Age	19 years
Social and family history	Student, lives with parents
Past medical history	Asthma
	Two previous admissions to intensive care for asthma
Current medication	Salbutamol
	Fluticasone propionate and salmeterol combined inhaler

BRAINSTORM

INSTRUCTIONS TO ROLE PLAYER (PATIENT)

NOT TO BE SEEN BY THE CANDIDATE

Patient background:

You are Mrs Protheroe, 19-year-old Thomas' mother.

You called the doctor for a home visit (panicking).

He has a sore throat and a fever.

You would like a home visit.

Opening statement:

'Hi Doctor, I want a home visit for my son.'

Freely divulged in response to open questions:

He has had a sore throat for 2 days.

He hasn't taken any over-the-counter drugs, except for lozenges.

He is alert and his breathing is fine.

Information divulged if asked specifically:

He isn't wheezing.

He isn't dribbling and has managed to eat some soup.

You don't think that he is well enough to talk to the doctor himself, his throat is too sore.

You refuse to let the doctor speak to him, despite the doctor's efforts.

The peak flow is 600 l/min (best is 620 l/min).

He also has a headache.

He doesn't have any neck stiffness or photophobia.

He is alert and his hands aren't cold.

You can't see a rash.

Your thermometer is broken but he feels hot.

He is laid up on the sofa and you don't feel that he is well enough to come to the surgery.

You are worried that, if he goes out of the house, he may catch a chill and develop a chest infection.

You understand that GPs are busy and you don't like to call the doctor out, but you don't want your son to travel.

You know how much GPs are paid and you feel that it's your right to have a visit.

You will complain to NHS England and newspapers if you don't get a visit.

NOTES

DATA-GATHERING, TECHNICAL AND ASSESSMENT SKILLS

- It is difficult to take a history over the phone.

- It is even more difficult when the history is taken from a third party.

- He is hot and, despite the unavailability of a thermometer, it is feasible that he has a fever.

- He has a sore throat and it is likely that he has an upper respiratory infection.

- The fact that Thomas is not dribbling is important, as dribbling could indicate significant upper respiratory disease that may require hospital management.

- He has a headache and evidence of meningism should be explored.

- He should be assessed for symptoms of sepsis.

- He has brittle asthma; one should ensure that he is not in respiratory distress.

CHAPTER 7

CLINICAL MANAGEMENT SKILLS

- Over-the-counter drugs (avoiding NSAIDs as he has brittle asthma) may be advised.

- Assessing him over the phone through a third party is difficult. Failure to visit and failure to examine are common causes for complaints against doctors. If you are unable to assess the patient adequately, and his mother refuses to bring him to the surgery, a home visit should be arranged.

- The GMC advises that a clinician should always justify their actions and adequately assess their patients (www.gmc-uk.org/guidance/good_medical_practice/GMC_GMP.pdf).

INTERPERSONAL SKILLS

- It would be helpful to explore why his mother is reluctant to bring her son to the surgery. Perhaps her ideas can be discussed and her concerns dealt with.

- A home visit may incur a delay in his care if there are other visits to deal with. He could be seen more quickly if she brought him in. By explaining this to her, she may be persuaded to bring him in.

- She has made life difficult by not allowing you to speak to her son. Irrespective of the legalities of consent, given that you have not been able to speak to him, you have a duty of care to the patient. If the patient is apparently too unwell to come to the surgery and you cannot persuade the mother to bring him in, you have little choice but to see him at home.

- Appropriate safety-netting should be discussed on the phone prior to arriving at the patient's house.

CASE 5

INSTRUCTIONS TO CANDIDATES (CASE NOTES)

Name	May Connolly
Age	79 years
Social and family history	Widowed
Past medical history	Moderate COPD
Current medication	Salbutamol prn
	Ipratoprium bromide qds
Additional info (results/letters)	FEV_1: 70% predicted

BRAINSTORM

INSTRUCTIONS TO ROLE PLAYER (PATIENT):

NOT TO BE SEEN BY THE CANDIDATE

Patient background:

You are May Connolly, you are 79 years old.

You live on your own.

You have lung disease due to smoking for 40 years of your life.

You no longer smoke.

You have been bleeding from your back passage for the last month.

Opening statement:

'I'm so embarrassed Doctor, I've been bleeding from my back passage.'

Freely divulged in response to open questions:

The blood tends to be mixed in with the stool.

You have had more diarrhoea lately, for about 3 months.

You have been experiencing mild abdominal pains in the right side of your 'stomach.'

You pressed on your abdomen yourself and felt a lump there.

Your weight is going down and you've felt tired lately.

You don't want to have any intimate examinations today.

You can't remember what your parents died from.

Information divulged if asked specifically:

You know in your heart you have cancer, but know little about the condition.

You want it confirmed so you can organise your will.

You would like to be referred to hospital for investigations, but you are worried about having surgery or chemotherapy.

Will these treatments be painful? Will you lose your hair and get infections? You know someone who had chemotherapy and they suffered with infections and ulcers in their mouth.

You aren't depressed or suicidal.

You have had a good life and you are not afraid to be with your husband, who died last year.

CHAPTER 7

NOTES

DATA-GATHERING, TECHNICAL AND ASSESSMENT SKILLS

- This patient has red flag symptoms suggestive of bowel malignancy. The following should be asked for in detail:
  - rectal bleeding in absence of anal symptoms
  - change in bowel habit especially to looser stool
  - weight loss
  - tenesmus
  - obstruction
  - palpable mass.
- Abdominal examination is essential in this situation, not only to confirm her own findings of a mass (assume that she has a malignant feeling mass for the purposes of this case; of course, the role player would not have positive clinical signs), but to assess its characteristics and check for hepatomegaly.
- A brief review of her conjunctivae would be reasonable as a gross sign of anaemia.
- Are there signs of acute bowel obstruction?
- She does not want a rectal examination and her wishes should be respected.

CLINICAL MANAGEMENT SKILLS

- A 2WW cancer referral is appropriate, if she agrees.
- This patient suspects that she has cancer. While it is likely, one should offer hope and explain that the diagnosis needs to be confirmed.
- Baseline bloods should be organised, in particular, full blood count. If she is anaemic, she should be commenced on iron supplements (you

shouldn't routinely commence iron replacement unless the aetiology of the anaemia is known). If required, Mrs Connolly may be amenable to having a blood transfusion as a day case or perhaps at a local hospice. Explain that you will contact her with the results.

- Her pain should be managed appropriately.

- Introduction to community cancer nurses would offer her support (once the diagnosis is confirmed).

- Explain the symptoms of bowel obstruction and what she should do if this arises, eg go to nearest Emergency Department or contact the practice immediately.

INTERPERSONAL SKILLS

- Agree that she is likely to have cancer, but explain that this will still need to be diagnosed in secondary care. What is her knowledge base? Does she know what bowel cancer is and what it means? What would she like to know? This will need to be done sensitively.

- Explore her concerns, in this case about treatment. If her fears of surgery are addressed, she may agree to have active treatment.

- Ensure that she is not depressed; she may refuse treatment as she wants to die. This isn't the case with this patient.

- Is she aware of the consequences of not having treatment? Unchecked spread of the condition, risk of bowel obstruction and death.

- Is she happy to be seen in hospital? Does she know what to expect? Does she know that she is not obliged to have any treatment if she doesn't want it?

- She should be made aware that she can change her mind about treatment any time.

FURTHER READING

The GMC has published guidance – *Consent: Patients and doctors making decisions together* which is relevant to many of the cases in general practice.

CHAPTER 7

SUMMARY OF *CONSENT: PATIENTS AND DOCTORS MAKING DECISIONS TOGETHER*

REVIEWED BY DR RAJ THAKKAR, GMC TODAY, MAY 2008

'Patient-centred consulting' dictates that we consider our patients' views and value their beliefs. By placing their illness in the context of their life and considering their ideas, concerns and expectations we enhance the patient experience.

The GMC's new guidance focuses on the principles of patient-centred consulting and emphasises working in partnership with patients. It's no surprise that many of the concepts described in the document are familiar to those versed in classic GP consulting models such as the one described in *The New Consultation* by Pendleton et al.

For some GPs, very little will change. After all, this is how many GPs consult routinely. More time may be needed with every patient to ensure that we gauge how much information they would like to know about their illness, take into account their health beliefs and finally inform them of the pros and cons of each treatment modality.

While intuition often tells us how much information a patient would like, patient-centred consulting dictates that one should explore this with the patient. Information should then be delivered with clarity, perhaps with the assistance of interpreters, diagrams and leaflets.

We must respect our patients' decisions, refrain from being judgemental and forge trusting professional relationships with them. Assessing capacity in line with the Mental Capacity Act 2005, managing patients who lack capacity and consent of those under the age of 18 are helpfully discussed in the guidance.

In order to make a decision about their treatment, patients need to be adequately informed about the condition itself, risks of not treating and the risks of each treatment. Doctors are therefore required to possess knowledge and hence keep up to date.

CHAPTER 7

Equally as important, skills are required to communicate the risks in ways that patients understand. While doctors should inform patients of risk, one has to maintain perspective and offer a balanced view. When explaining serious risks, one ought to present the likelihood of the adverse event occurring, what symptoms and signs to be aware of, and management and prognosis of the adverse outcome.

Scaring our patients, however, may only act to confuse and perhaps inadvertently dissuade them from accepting vital treatment. Doctors should, nevertheless, respect their patients' treatment choice, even if it is not in their best medical interest, so long as they are of sound mind.

The GMC's guidance acts to empower patients and deliver a more satisfying service. Doctors are obliged to embrace it, move with the times and provide a robust and first-class service.

Reproduced with kind permission of the GMC.

CASE 6

INSTRUCTIONS TO CANDIDATES (CASE NOTES)

You are a locum doctor at a busy practice

Name   Sarah Mullen

Age   37 years

Address   11 Archway Road

                                        Marble Hill

Social and family history   Married

Past medical history   Nil

Last entry 6 months ago (practice nurse):

                                        Smear taken

                                        Full sweep

                                        Cervix visualised

Result:

Severe dyskaryosis – normal, no action

BRAINSTORM

INSTRUCTIONS TO ROLE PLAYER (PATIENT)

NOT TO BE SEEN BY THE CANDIDATE

Patient background:

You are Sarah Mullen and you are 37 years old.

You have been suffering from unusual vaginal bleeding and are very worried.

You are a secretary at the local factory.

Opening statement:

'Hello Doctor, I'm a little worried, I've been bleeding.'

Freely divulged in response to open questions:

You live with your husband and are in a happy and committed relationship.

You don't have children but you're hoping to try soon.

You have noticed abnormal vaginal bleeding for the last 3 months.

It has been getting worse recently and you have noticed some blood clots.

You have noticed bleeding in between periods and also after sexual intercourse.

Information divulged if asked specifically:

Your last smear was 6 months ago. You thought nothing of the bleeding initially as you thought your smear was normal.

You understood the surgery's policy was to contact patients if smears were abnormal.

As the symptoms persisted, you thought that you should get checked out.

You would like to double-check whether the results of the smear were normal.

When you learn about the abnormal result, you would like to know why you weren't informed.

You want to know how this will affect your fertility and what the cause of the bleeding is likely to be.

You would like to know what the practice is going to do about the situation.

You would rather not have an examination today.

You would like a referral to a gynaecologist: you have private insurance.

NOTES

DATA-GATHERING, TECHNICAL AND ASSESSMENT SKILLS

- A detailed menstrual history is essential.
- Does she have any red flag symptoms suggesting malignancy?
- It is helpful to establish exactly where she had her smear done and by whom.
- Has she moved and has the practice got her right address?
- Was there any evidence in the notes that any action was taken on the abnormal smear result?

CLINICAL MANAGEMENT SKILLS

- This patient shows concerning symptoms.
- She ought to have a full blood count.
- The most important act is to exclude a gynaecological malignancy.
- Organising a quick referral letter to her private consultant is appropriate.

CHAPTER 7

INTERPERSONAL SKILLS

- Her wishes regarding examination should be respected.

- What are her ideas and concerns? Does she have any idea that this may represent a malignancy?

- She has private insurance and a referral to a gynaecologist is indicated. Does she have a specialist in mind, or would she like a recommendation? Does she know the process of how to organise a private referral? For example, she will have to ring her insurance company to obtain an authorisation code, and also contact the private hospital to organise an appointment.

- It is likely that she will be angry and upset.

- Does she have any views on what she would like you to do? She may not want to take the matter further, or she may make a complaint or even bring legal action against the practice.

- It will be difficult as a locum to resolve the situation. Tell the patient that you will bring it to the attention of the partners and practice manager. A full investigation (significant event analysis) should be held.

FURTHER READING

Chambers R. *How to... Learn from significant events*, 2010. www.GPonline. com, 2010.

CASE 7

INSTRUCTIONS TO CANDIDATES (CASE NOTES)

You are new to the practice; it is your first day as a salaried doctor.

Name	Perry Smith
Age	61 years
Social and family history	Married, four children
Past medical history	MI 3 years ago
Current medication	Aspirin 75 mg od
	Ramipril 10 mg od
	Simvastatin 40 mg nocte
	Atenolol 100 mg od
	Tadalafil 10 mg prn

Last entry in notes:

'Invite patient to come in to discuss meds. He should not have been getting tadalafil on NHS. Need to prescribe privately only. Doesn't fulfil "SLS" criteria'

BRAINSTORM

INSTRUCTIONS TO ROLE PLAYER (PATIENT)

NOT TO BE SEEN BY THE CANDIDATE

Patient background:

You are Perry Smith, you are 61 years old.

You are a carpenter, although business hasn't been good recently.

You have no idea what the issue is regarding your medication.

You are shocked and upset when the doctor says that you need to pay for your tadalafil.

You have been taking them since your heart attack.

Opening statement:

'Hi Doctor, I've not met you before, my old doctor has retired. I've been asked to come in to discuss my tablets.'

Freely divulged in response to open questions:

It transformed your marriage which is brilliant at the moment. Prior to the tablets, your erectile dysfunction was seriously affecting your relationship.

You use about 2 tablets a week.

You wonder what do other men do, and how can you get them for free?

Information divulged if asked specifically:

You don't understand why you got them for free up until now.

You are over 60 and think you're entitled to free prescriptions.

You can't afford to pay for them.

If you don't have them it will destroy your marriage and you will get depressed.

You want to know how this could have happened.

What practice systems are in place to ensure that this doesn't happen?

You have heard that you can buy them over the internet; you wonder what the doctor's views are on this.

CHAPTER 7

You would like the practice to pay some of the prescription as a gesture of good will.

You would like to know if there anything else that could help with erectile dysfunction.

You don't suffer any chest pain when you exert yourself.

You don't have a tremor.

You have a good urine flow.

You have a good sex drive.

Your nipples don't leak fluid.

You don't have to get up in the night to pass urine and your weight is stable.

You are happy, although you have a few financial pressures.

You drink half a bottle of wine per night. No more on weekends.

You don't smoke.

You don't exercise.

NOTES

DATA-GATHERING, TECHNICAL AND ASSESSMENT SKILLS

- Establish his use of tadalafil, eg two tablets/week.

- Understand his knowledge of the current NHS prescribing guidelines with respect to phosphodiesterase inhibitors for erectile dysfunction.

- Does he have any symptoms suggestive of conditions entitling him to free tadalafil?

- Was he ever checked for causes of erectile dysfunction by his previous GP?

Tip

✓ **Make use of the BNF in this consultation – it will list those entitled to free tadalafil. These include:**

   ✓ **those receiving the drug before 14 February 1998**

   ✓ **those suffering from:**

      ✓ **diabetes**

      ✓ **multiple sclerosis**

      ✓ **Parkinson's disease**

      ✓ **polio**

      ✓ **prostate cancer**

      ✓ **severe pelvic injury**

      ✓ **single gene neurological disease**

      ✓ **spina bifida**

      ✓ **spinal cord injury**

      ✓ **patients having dialysis or having received a renal transplant for renal failure**

      ✓ **previous prostatectomy or radical pelvic surgery.**

- Consider other causes of erectile dysfunction in the history.

- How much alcohol does he drink? This may be contributing to his erectile dysfunction? Is he aware if this?

- Is he depressed?

- Does he have symptoms of prostatism, diabetes or thyroid disease?

- Does he have low libido? Does he have galactorrhoea (prolactinoma)?

CLINICAL MANAGEMENT SKILLS

- It may be reasonable to change his atenolol to a cardioselective β blocker or to reduce his atenolol to a lower dose. This may be the underlying cause of his erectile dysfunction. His pulse and blood pressure should be checked and he should be warned about unmasking angina if his β blockers are altered.

- Discuss a reduction in alcohol as a form of treatment.

- Exercise should be encouraged, although he should be warned about angina.

- Arranging a series of baseline bloods (FBC, glucose, prolactin, testosterone, TFTs, PSA) and the use of a depression screening tool may appropriate.

- Consider psychosexual counselling as a therapy.

INTERPERSONAL SKILLS

- This is a difficult case to manage on your first day.

- You have to break it to him that he has to pay for his drugs. This should be done sensitively.

- Giving him options about improving his erectile dysfunction may give him hope and pacify him, eg reducing or changing his atenolol and changing his lifestyle. Other options would be to check him for underlying causes such as diabetes and prostate disease. Once given options, he should feel enabled to choose what suits him.

- It is a mistake by the practice, and admitting this was a regrettable oversight is not unreasonable.

- The practice cannot pay for his drugs.

CHAPTER 7

- Explaining the system to him, and perhaps suggesting that he was fortunate to have received free tadalafil up until now, may make him see the positive side of the situation. This could come across in an aggressive tone and you should be careful to say it in a passive tone.

- Explaining that all patients in the practice, who have been inappropriately prescribed tadalafil free on the NHS, have been contacted may make him feel less victimised.

- You may offer to carry out a significant event analysis and write to him with the outcome.

- Appropriate follow-up reviewing the results of your action plan (including to check if he is experiencing angina) is essential.

CHAPTER 7

CASE 8

INSTRUCTIONS TO CANDIDATES (CASE NOTES)

You have never met this patient before.

Name	Elizabeth Ross
Age	49 years
Social and family history	Store manager
Past medical history	Depression
Current medication	Citalopram 20 mg od

BRAINSTORM

INSTRUCTIONS TO ROLE PLAYER (PATIENT)

NOT TO BE SEEN BY THE CANDIDATE

Patient background:

You are Elizabeth Ross, you are 49 years old.

You have depression.

You have run out of antidepressant tablets.

You normally get a month's worth at a time.

You have been taking citalopram for 8 months ever since your husband admitted that he was having an affair. You are still with him and things between you are slowly improving.

Opening statement:

'I've come to get my tablets Doctor.'

Freely divulged in response to open questions:

You haven't taken your tablets for 5 days as you think that you may be getting side effects. You don't feel that you have any withdrawal effects.

You sleep until 7 am, but you find it difficult to get off to sleep.

Your concentration and memory aren't what they should be and you feel that it's impacting your performance at work.

You are eating well and your weight is stable. Your mood is worse in the mornings.

Information divulged if asked specifically:

You and your partner are starting to have a physical relationship again. You haven't been able to reach orgasm and you think that may be due to the tablets, but you are very embarrassed to ask about that.

You feel guilty that you haven't fully forgiven your partner.

He never hits you.

You would like to stay with him and are sure that the future is promising; you are just not there yet. You are not suicidal.

You don't think citalopram is right for you; you feel emotionally numbed and would like to have counselling, you have heard counselling is very effective.

You have been drinking more alcohol lately, to help with you sleep. You don't have panic attacks or obsessional thoughts, although you sometimes think about your partner with another woman. You are a little anxious but it's not that bad at the moment.

You haven't been drinking this much for long and you know it's wrong. You feel bad about drinking this much. You drink a 750 ml bottle of 12% wine per night. You think each bottle has 5 units but you are not sure. You only drink in the evenings and never drink and drive. Your partner hasn't commented on your drinking.

NOTES

DATA-GATHERING, TECHNICAL AND ASSESSMENT SKILLS

- It is important to establish the background to her depression and what her current symptoms are. Check for biological (sleep disturbance, diurnal-mood variation, concentration and memory disturbance, loss of libido), cognitive (guilt, poor outlook for the future, low self-esteem, anxiety, suicidal ideation), and if appropriate psychotic (auditory hallucinations, delusions) features.

- You may want to use a validated questionnaire, if available, such as the Hospital Anxiety and Depression (HAD) score – evidence suggests questionnaires such as this have a very good negative predictive value.

- A suicidal risk assessment is important.

- Does she feel that she is improving or getting worse? If not, why not?

- How is she managing with her tablets? Is she taking them regularly? Does she have any side effects?

CHAPTER 7

$$\text{Units} = \frac{\text{volume of alcohol she drinks}}{1000} \times \% \text{ alcohol}$$

$$= \frac{750}{1000} \times 12$$

$$= 9 \text{ units/day}$$

$$= 63 \text{ units per week}$$

Fig. 11 Volume of alcohol consumed

- Establish how much alcohol she is actually drinking. This can be done using the formula in Figure 11.

- How is her situation affecting her quality of life?

CLINICAL MANAGEMENT SKILLS

- She hasn't taken citalopram for 5 days. As she isn't keen on continuing the course, it is reasonable to not to prescribe any more (unless she is getting withdrawal effects).

- She would like counselling – a referral should be made. Counselling would address depression and alcohol use. Has she considered relationship counselling?

- Consider prescribing vitamin B supplements.

- Does she need time off work?

- Is she interested in self-help books or websites? Would she prefer over-the-counter, rather than prescribed, therapy, eg St John's wort.

- Regular follow-up is imperative.

INTERPERSONAL SKILLS

- Sensitivity is crucial to gaining her trust. She must feel supported.

- How would she best like to be helped? Offer her options, eg changing antidepressants, counselling. Does she know what to expect from different treatment modalities, what they entail and how long it may take for them to work?

- Many people are embarrassed when discussing sexual matters. If she offers a cue, one approach would be to say some women have sexual problems on citalopram and ask if that applies to her.

CASE 9

INSTRUCTIONS TO CANDIDATES (CASE NOTES)

Name	Jessica Ronson
Age	26 years
Social and family history	Married, one child, 5 years old
Past medical history	Anxiety

Tip

✓ Be aware the past medical history may not bear any relationship to the presenting case.

BRAINSTORM

INSTRUCTIONS TO ROLE PLAYER (PATIENT)

NOT TO BE SEEN BY THE CANDIDATE

Patient background:

You are Jessica Ronson, you are 26 years old.

You have a history of anxiety but your symptoms are under control.

You are worried about your son, Alfie. Alfie is normally well.

One of his classmates was diagnosed with meningitis 2 weeks ago. She will be fine and the children in her class, including Alfie, were given the all clear by Public Health.

Opening statement:

'Hi Doctor, I need to know about meningitis.'

Freely divulged in response to open questions:

You are confused about how meningitis may present.

Information divulged if asked specifically:

You heard someone say; if he doesn't have a rash it means he doesn't have meningitis, but one of the mums at school said that was wrong.

You are sure that people with meningitis also have a headache.

You have heard that the vaccination won't fully protect him against meningitis. You would like to know if that's true and why?

NOTES

DATA-GATHERING, TECHNICAL AND ASSESSMENT SKILLS

- Finding out what happened to Alfie's classmate would be a good starting point.

- Has he had his meningitis C vaccination?

- You may want to check his medical history: Is he immunocompromised, eg splenectomy?

- What does she understand about meningococcal disease?

CLINICAL MANAGEMENT SKILLS

- Much of this consultation will revolve around delivering information in a way that she understands.

- The description of meningitis, septicaemia and the differences between the two conditions should be discussed.

- In particular, the misunderstanding that the absence of a rash excludes a diagnosis of meningitis should be explored.

- A more general discussion about what to watch out for in a sick child of any cause is relevant.

INTERPERSONAL SKILLS

- What is her level of knowledge? There is little point in telling her what she already knows.

- Consider if she has any particular questions, or would she like you to tell her about meningitis in general?

- When discussing features of meningococcal disease, you should check that she understands what you mean, in order to achieve shared understanding.

- Have you relieved her fears?

Tip

 ✓ **Check that you understand the patient and the patient understands you**

- She shouldn't be made to feel ignorant and should be given the opportunity to ask questions.

- Offering a leaflet about the features of meningitis and meningococcal septicaemia will help reiterate what you have said.

Tip

 ✓ **Don't say that you will give her a leaflet at the end of the consultation, because you may not have one in the surgery during the exam. Say that you will send her one in the post, give her a web page (as long as she's on the net) or suggest that she picks one up from reception.**

- Suggest that she can give you a call at the surgery if she has further questions.

- You may offer to arrange an evening meeting at the local school to discuss meningitis with parents and teachers.

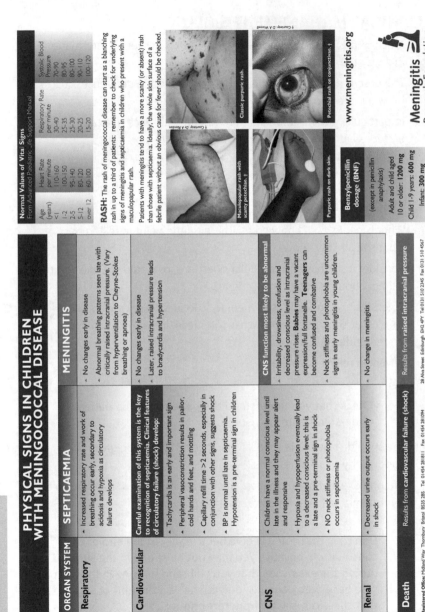

PHYSICAL SIGNS IN CHILDREN WITH MENINGOCOCCAL DISEASE

ORGAN SYSTEM	SEPTICAEMIA	MENINGITIS
Respiratory	⁃ Increased respiratory rate and work of breathing occur early, secondary to acidosis and hypoxia as circulatory failure develops	⁃ No changes early in disease ⁃ Abnormal breathing patterns seen late with critically raised intracranial pressure. (Vary from hyperventilation to Cheyne-Stokes breathing or apnoea)
Cardiovascular	**Careful examination of this system is the key to recognition of septicaemia. Clinical features of circulatory failure (shock) develop:** ⁃ Tachycardia is an early and important sign ⁃ Peripheral vasoconstriction results in pallor, cold hands and feet, and mottling ⁃ Capillary refill time >2 seconds, especially in conjunction with other signs, suggests shock ⁃ BP is normal until late in septicaemia. ⁃ Hypotension is a pre-terminal sign in children	⁃ No changes early in disease ⁃ Later, raised intracranial pressure leads to bradycardia and hypertension
CNS	⁃ Children have a normal conscious level until late in the illness and they may appear alert and responsive ⁃ Hypoxia and hypoperfusion eventually lead to a decreased conscious level: this is a late and a pre-terminal sign in shock ⁃ NO neck stiffness or photophobia occurs in septicaemia	**CNS function most likely to be abnormal** ⁃ Irritability, drowsiness, confusion and decreased conscious level as intracranial pressure rises. **Babies** may have a vacant expression/full fontanelle. **Teenagers** can become confused and combative ⁃ Neck stiffness and photophobia are uncommon signs in early meningitis in young children.
Renal	⁃ Decreased urine output occurs early in shock	⁃ No change in meningitis
Death	Results from **cardiovascular failure (shock)**	Results from **raised intracranial pressure**

Normal Values of Vital Signs
From Advanced Paediatric Life Support Manual

Age (years)	Heart Rate per minute	Respiratory Rate per minute	Systolic Blood Pressure
<1	110-160	30-40	70-90
1-2	100-150	25-35	80-95
2-5	95-40	25-30	80-100
5-12	80-120	20-25	90-110
over 12	60-100	15-20	100-120

RASH: The rash of meningococcal disease can start as a blanching rash in up to a third of patients: remember to check for underlying signs of meningitis and septicaemia in children who present with a maculopapular rash.

Patients with meningitis tend to have a more scanty (or absent) rash than those with septicaema. Ideally, the whole skin surface of a febrile patient without an obvious cause for fever should be checked.

† Courtesy: Dr A Riordan

Maculopapular rash with scanty petechiae. †

Purpuric rash on dark skin.

Classic purpuric rash.

Petechial rash on conjunctivae. †

† Courtesy: D A Warrell

www.meningitis.org

Benzylpenicillin dosage (BNF)

(except in penicillin anaphylaxis)

Adult and child aged 10 or older: **1200 mg**
Child 1-9 years: **600 mg**
Infant: **300 mg**

Meningitis Research Foundation

Registered Office: Midland Way, Thornbury, Bristol BS35 2BS   Tel 01454 281811   Fax 01454 281094   28 Alva Street, Edinburgh EH2 4PY Tel 0131 510 2345   Fax 0131 510 4567
71 Botanic Avenue, Belfast BT7 1JL   Tel 028 9032 1283   Fax 028 9032 1284   Office also in the Republic of Ireland
Offices: Belfast, Bristol, Dublin, Edinburgh. A charity registered in England and Wales no 1091105. In Scotland no SC037586 & in Ireland CHY 12030.   © Meningitis Research Foundation 08/2011   05dUK   7th Edition

Fig. 12 Meningitis Research Foundation – Physical Signs in Children with Meningococcal Disease. Reproduced with kind permission.

SIGNS TO LOOK OUT FOR IN MENINGITIS: RAPID DIAGNOSIS AND TREATMENT OF MENINGOCOCCAL DISEASE IS VITAL

Meningococcal disease is the leading infectious cause of childhood death in the UK. Around half of cases occur in children aged 4 years or under, although peaks are seen in teenagers and elderly people.

There are at least 13 different serotypes of *Neisseria meningitidis*, the causative agent, although most cases of meningococcal disease in the UK are caused by B or C strains. Introduction of the MenC vaccine in 1999 resulted in a marked decrease in the number of cases.

Meningococcal disease may cause septicaemia, meningitis or both. The organism may also cause arthritis, osteomyelitis or ophthalmic complications.

The early stages of meningococcal disease may present as non-specific flu-like symptoms so it is important to look for signs of septicaemia or meningitis in all febrile patients without obvious infection.

MENINGOCOCCAL SEPTICAEMIA

Meningococcal septicaemia is an emergency and is fatal in around 20 per cent of cases. A high index of suspicion and thorough examination are required when children present with signs of septicaemia.

A diagnostic tool such as the Glasgow meningococcal septicaemia prognostic score can help identify those children requiring immediate emergency treatment.

Bacterial death in the blood triggers a massive inflammatory reaction with failure of the endothelium and the clotting cascade. This produces the classic non-blanching purpuric rash of meningococcal septicaemia. In up to a third of cases the rash is maculopapular.

CHAPTER 7

Early symptoms include tachycardia, increased respiratory rate and peripheral vasoconstriction. Other features include hypoxia and oliguria. Abdominal pain, sometimes with diarrhoea, may be present and joint and bone pains can be severe.

The peripheries may be cool and mottled. A capillary refill time greater than 2 seconds on the sternum or forehead is abnormal while one of 4 seconds or more in the peripheries is suggestive of shock.

Hypotension and altered consciousness are late signs in children. Without treatment, organ failure and cardiovascular collapse will eventually lead to death in these cases.

MENINGITIS

Meningitis has a different presentation to septicaemia and a much lower mortality rate at less than 5 per cent.

Symptoms include severe headache, impaired consciousness, photophobia and neck stiffness, although in young children both neck stiffness and photophobia occur later in the illness and up to a third do not even develop neck stiffness.

Kernig's sign may be positive. Babies may also present with a tense fontanelle, vacant stare, high-pitched cry, poor feeding or a change in tone.

In older children and teenagers meningitis can cause changes in behaviour such as confusion or aggression. These signs are sometimes presumed to be alcohol related.

Meningitis may also cause raised intracranial pressure, which can eventually lead to cardiorespiratory compromise and death.

Signs of this include: declining consciousness; unequal, dilated or poorly responsive pupils; hypertension; and relative bradycardia.

IMMEDIATE CARE

A child presenting with meningitis or a fever and purpuric rash should be treated for meningococcal disease without delay. Blood tests to confirm the infection can be carried out after antibiotics have been administered.

Antibiotics should be given intravenously where possible. Benzylpenicillin and cefotaxime are first-line agents.

Chloramphenicol may be used if there is a definite history of allergy to these agents. Oxygen should be given.

Treatment for sepsis may also include fluid resuscitation and inotropic support, usually within a hospital setting.

A lumbar puncture should be taken when meningitis is suspected. Treatment should also be administered where the diagnosis is unclear.

A child with worrying symptoms should be transferred to a paediatric unit via a blue-light ambulance, with a receiving team on standby.

NOTIFICATION

Meningococcal disease is a notifiable disease. The consultant in communicable disease control is responsible for ensuring that anyone who has been in close contact with the patient receives prophylaxis.

Drugs used to clear carriage include rifampicin, ciprofloxacin and ceftriaxone.

Contacts should be informed that these drugs are not used to treat infection and the signs of established meningococcal disease should be discussed with them.

By Dr R Thakkar

Reproduced with the kind permission of *Haymarket Medical*, April 2008

CHAPTER 7

CASE 10: HOME VISIT

INSTRUCTIONS TO CANDIDATES (CASE NOTES)

You arrive at this patient's home. She requested a home visit for abdominal pain. You have a paper summary of her notes with you. Her grandson lets you into the house.

You have a doctor's bag with standard equipment and drugs (including opiates).

Name	Mary Baron
Age	72 years
Social and family history	Lives with grandson (age 17), recently widowed
Past medical history	MI × 3
	Rheumatoid arthritis
	Depression
Current medication	Aspirin 75 mg od
	Ramipril 10 mg od
	Simvastatin 40 mg nocte
	Atenolol 50 mg od
	Paracetamol 1g qds
	Tramadol 50 mg qds
	Prednisolone 5 mg od
	Methotrexate 10 mg weekly
	Alendronic acid 70 mg weekly
	Folic acid 5 mg weekly
	Ibuprofen 400 mg prn
	Fluoxetine 20 mg od

BRAINSTORM

EXAMINATION FINDINGS

Information offered on iPad if appropriate

Pulse 110/min, BP 109/40
Sweaty and has a rigid abdomen.

INSTRUCTIONS TO ROLE PLAYER (PATIENT)

NOT TO BE SEEN BY THE CANDIDATE

Patient background:

You are Mary Baron, you are 72 years old.

You have severe abdominal pain.

It started suddenly about 3 hours ago.

Opening statement:

'Doctor, help me, I'm in pain.'

Freely divulged in response to open questions:

It is above your belly button.

You have been vomiting.

You can't move because you're in too much pain.

You don't have any chest pain.

This is the worst pain you have ever experienced.

Information divulged if asked specifically:

You don't have any drug allergies.

You are scared to go into hospital; you don't want to get MRSA. You agree to go when the doctor recommends it.

You are sweaty and your heart is pounding fast in your chest.

Whenever the doctor examines your stomach, it is exquisitely painful and feels rock hard.

You can't stand the pain any more.

You think that you may be having a heart attack.

NOTES

DATA-GATHERING, TECHNICAL AND ASSESSMENT SKILLS

- It is likely that this patient has a perforated peptic ulcer. She takes a number of drugs that put her at risk for peptic ulcer disease.

- As she is unwell, it is reasonable to take a quick and directed history.

- Her vital signs should be measured: temperature, pulse and blood pressure.

- Examination of her abdomen would reveal a rigid abdomen with guarding (the examiner may well hand you the examination findings).

- Ask about chest pain, particularly given her history of coronary artery disease.

CLINICAL MANAGEMENT SKILLS

- It is clear that this patient needs a surgical opinion.

- It would be appropriate to call 999.

- If she is not allergic to any medication, intramuscular/intravenous opiates and antiemetics should be given.

Tip

✓ You should not administer any drugs during the CSA.

- The surgical team at the local hospital should be notified that you are sending the patient in.

- You will have to write a letter of referral to the surgical team.

- You should wait for the ambulance to arrive; she is at risk of cardiac arrest (you would have to express that you would wait for the ambulance to the examiner).

CHAPTER 7

INTERPERSONAL SKILLS

- Both the patient and her grandson will be worried and concerned.

- Is she happy for her grandson to be present while you are talking to her?

- You will need to gain her confidence, keep cool and demonstrate that you are in control.

- Even though she requires hospital management, it is important to keep her informed as to what you think is going on and why you think she requires hospital treatment.

- It would be reasonable if you ask if she has any concerns with your plan to arrange hospital management. Her concerns should be addressed and expectations discussed. This may relieve her anxiety. In addition to contracting MRSA and having a 'heart attack' she may be concerned about dying, never coming out of hospital and what may happen to her in hospital.

CASE 11

INSTRUCTIONS TO CANDIDATES (CASE NOTES)

Name   Hilary Gilligan

Age   69 years

Social and family history   Married, five children

Past medical history   Shingles × 2

Current medication   Nil

Previous consultation (one week ago):

Shingles, has had two previous episodes this year.

Right T10, for aciclovir.

Review if concerned.

BRAINSTORM

INSTRUCTIONS TO ROLE PLAYER (PATIENT)

NOT TO BE SEEN BY THE CANDIDATE

Patient background:

You are Hilary Gilligan, 69 years old.

You have shingles, diagnosed last week by another doctor at your practice.

Opening statement:

'Hi Doctor, I need your advice.'

Freely divulged in response to open questions:

You are worried because your daughter is pregnant and you think that you may give her shingles if you see her.

She is 7 weeks' pregnant.

Information divulged if asked specifically:

She had chickenpox when she was a child.

You think that shingles is caught from other people with shingles.

You know that there is a link between chickenpox and shingles, but you don't fully understand it.

You would like to know more about shingles.

This is your third episode of shingles this year.

You have had some weight loss and night sweats lately.

You are not stressed and can't wait to see your first grandchild.

You have been more tired lately.

Your bowel habit hasn't changed although you have had some abdominal pain.

You haven't had any bone pain.

NOTES

DATA-GATHERING, TECHNICAL AND ASSESSMENT SKILLS

- This consultation has two issues. The first focuses on the behaviour of the herpes zoster virus. The second is about the management of a patient with potential immunoparesis.

- Regarding her recurrent shingles, you should consider immunoparesis. Given her age group, conditions such as CLL, lymphoma, myeloma, myelodysplasia, marrow infiltration and diabetes should be considered.

- Red flag symptoms should be sought.

- Examination of her abdomen to check for hepatosplenomegaly and lymphadenopathy shows forward and lateral thinking.

Tip

✓ Explain why you are asking questions and what you are examining for. 'Sign-posting' to the patient would help her understand your thought process. For example, she may find it odd if, out of the blue, you expressed the wish to examine her abdomen when she was concerned about her daughter getting shingles. If you discussed that some patients with recurrent shingles have an enlarged spleen and you were just checking hers, she would think that you are a thoughtful doctor.

CLINICAL MANAGEMENT SKILLS

- Check FBC (film for smear cells and CLL), ESR, myeloma screen, glucose. Chest radiograph for mediastinal lymph nodes. You are looking for conditions predisposing her to recurrent shingles.

INTERPERSONAL SKILLS

- It is helpful to know what the patient's current level of understanding about chickenpox and shingles is. Once this is clear, you can offer an explanation clarifying any deficiencies in her knowledge base, which is:

  - Chickenpox occurs in patients who have never been exposed to the herpes zoster virus (by exposure to chickenpox or shingles). It is unusual to get chickenpox more than once.

  - Once a patient has had chickenpox, the virus sits dormant in the spinal cord (dorsal root ganglion).

  - For many reasons, the virus can reactivate and migrate along a (sensory) nerve to cause shingles in the distribution of that nerve (dermatomal).

  - A patient with shingles can shed the (herpes zoster) virus and cause chickenpox in someone who has never had chicken pox before.

  - Pregnant women who have never had chickenpox before are at risk.

- She should not be made to feel silly.

- Checking her understanding by summarising what you have said is important.

- What are her ideas on patients who have recurrent shingles? Does she know that there may be underlying causes?

- A leaflet on shingles and chickenpox, perhaps from www.patient.co.uk, would back up what you have said.

- She should be followed up to discuss her blood tests.

CHAPTER 7

CASE 12

INSTRUCTIONS TO CANDIDATES (CASE NOTES)

Name	Mary Smith
Age	63 years
Social and family history	Married, three children
Past medical history	OA
	Hypothyroidism
	Obesity
	Hypertension
Current medication	Paracetamol 1 g qds
	Amlodipine 5 mg od
	Levothyroxine 150 mcg od

Last consultation (one week ago):

Nocturia, polydypsia and weight loss. BP persistently raised > 150/90.

Plan – Check fasting blood sugar, TSH and BP with nurse, then review next week

Additional info (results/letters)

Glucose	16.7 mmol/l
TSH	Euthyroid
BP (with nurse)	122/73

BRAINSTORM

INSTRUCTIONS TO ROLE PLAYER (PATIENT)

NOT TO BE SEEN BY THE CANDIDATE

Patient background:

You are Mary Smith, you are 63 years old.

You live with your husband, who is disabled after his stroke last year, and your youngest son who has recently finished his university degree.

You have osteoarthritis.

You have had hypothyroidism for 15 years. It runs in the family, both you mother and your sister have it.

You have been losing weight recently which you were pleased about. However, you also noticed you were drinking more than normal and passing a lot of urine.

Opening statement:

'I've come to get my results Doctor!'

Freely divulged in response to open questions:

You have been more tired recently, which you don't quite understand. Last time, when your levothyroxine dose was too high, you didn't suffer fatigue.

Your bowel habit is normal and you're not sensitive to extremes of temperature.

You try to eat healthily to help control your blood pressure which has been hard to control.

You don't smoke.

Information divulged if asked specifically:

You are concerned that your levothyroxine dose isn't right.

Once you were given the diagnosis of diabetes you become concerned about having to check your blood sugars every day and having to inject yourself with insulin. You don't know exactly what diabetes is or what the complications are.

NOTES

DATA-GATHERING, TECHNICAL AND ASSESSMENT SKILLS

- This patient has type 2 diabetes. She is symptomatic with a raised fasting blood sugar above 7.0 mmol/l. Had she been asymptomatic, she would require a further confirmatory test.

- Much of the consultation will revolve around educating the patient.

- It would be helpful to confirm the history and to consider what her concerns are. You can then break the bad news bearing in mind her health beliefs. Many patients are fearful of being diabetic.

- Features of diabetes itself should be asked for: polyuria, polydypsia, weight loss and fatigue.

- She should be asked about any symptoms of cardiovascular, eye and neuropathic disease.

- You should discuss lifestyle, does she smoke, what is her diet like, does she exercise?

- It is important to check her blood pressure.

CLINICAL MANAGEMENT SKILLS

- Holistic and systematic care of diabetic patients is essential. Most practices will have a diabetes clinic and may have a doctor and/or a nurse who takes a special interest in the subject.

Tip

   ✓ **You won't be able to discuss all the issues related to diabetes in 10 minutes. Just go with the patient's agenda and her immediate concerns, and organise an appointment with the diabetes nurse in the practice diabetes clinic.**

- Are there any diabetes patient groups locally and would she like to attend?

CHAPTER 7

411

- She should be put on the diabetes register and be recalled for regular review.

- Lifestyle is a major part of diabetes management. It is important to impress on her the importance of losing weight and how this may benefit her arthritis as well as her diabetes.

- Further bloods are required: HbA1c, U&Es and fasting lipids, with appropriate follow-up for further management. Note HbA1c should be used to diagnose diabetes, rather than a fasting glucose.

- The nurse should weigh her and repeat her blood pressure when she takes her blood.

- Urinary albumin:creatinine ratio (ACR) is required. She should be asked to drop a first-pass (rather than mid-stream) urine sample into the practice. Does she know why you are checking her urine?

- She may be commenced on a statin as evidence suggests that diabetic patients are at as much risk of ischaemic cardiac events as patients who have an established diagnosis of coronary artery disease.

- Blood pressure should be appropriately controlled in diabetes.

Tip

   ✓   **Use the BNF or MIMS (if available) during the consultation as you would in a routine surgery. They often give useful clinical pointers and guidelines if you're stuck!**

- She should be referred to the retinopathy clinic for regular assessment. Explain why this is important and check out whether she is happy for you to go ahead with the referral.

CHAPTER 7

INTERPERSONAL SKILLS

- Explaining a new diagnosis of diabetes brings with it a raft of issues, many of which have been discussed earlier. You won't be able to discuss all of the issues in a 10-minute consultation. It is far better to concentrate on a few major points, so that she feels satisfied and empowered, than to deliver a unilateral speech on diabetes, leaving her feeling overwhelmed.

- What does she think diabetes is? Does she know why people get it? Does she understand why it is important to treat it properly?

- For many people, diabetes is a mystery while others are well aware of its complications. It is important to assess what her level of knowledge is and to pitch your consultation accordingly. She should be educated as much as possible.

- What are her concerns? Insulin dependence is a common concern.

- She may become upset and sensitivity should be demonstrated.

- It is important to get her on board with treatment in order to optimise her care.

- Can you offer any leaflets or websites if she has access to the internet?

- Follow-up is important; she is likely to have many more questions once she leaves your consulting room and you will need to discuss the results of the investigations that you have arranged. You may want to offer a double (20-minute) appointment next time and ask her to write down any questions that she may have.

KEY:
a Or individually agreed target
b Consider prandial glucose regulator if patient has erratic lifestyle
c Continue DPP4 inhibitor or glitazone only if HbA$_{1c}$ declines by ≥0.5% in six months

Fig. 13 Management of type 2 diabetes, NICE 2009.

Reproduced with the kind permission of MIMS

KEY POINTS – NICE, TYPE 2 DIABETES

- Self-monitoring and education important
- Patient-centred care
- Dietary and lifestyle advice
    - eg smoking, exercise
    - advise low GI foods, oily fish, reduce dairy products
- When initiating insulin the following are important: education, telephone support, self-monitoring and management of hypoglycaemic episodes
- Be sensitive to patients' cultural, linguistic, cognitive needs
- HbA1c general target 6.5% or less
- Target may be higher based on discussion with individual
- Monitor HbA1c 2–6 monthly if sugars unstable or 6 monthly if stable
- Self-monitoring for all patients, if they are able, unless they are just controlled on diet or metformin
- Advise self-monitoring of glucose to assess safety, eg when driving
- Patients should have an overall management plan.

METFORMIN

- Increase dose over a few weeks – minimises GI side effects
- Care if creatinine > 130 μmol/L or eGFR < 45 ml/min
- Stop if creatinine > 150 μmol/L or eGFR < 30 ml/min
- BMJ, 2007 – metformin does not, on its own, cause lactic acidosis.

SULFONYLUREA

- Warn about hypoglycaemia.

CHAPTER 7

415

GLITAZONES

- Diabetes Care, 2007 – increased risk of heart failure.

BLOOD PRESSURE MANAGEMENT

- If end-organ damage, aim for BP < 130/80 mmHg, otherwise < 140/80 mmHg. The British Hypertension Society recommends < 130/80 mmHg generally for diabetes
- If not hypertensive and no renal disease, review annually
- If BP > 150/90 mmHg repeat in 1 month
- If BP > 130/80 (if end-organ damage) or > 140/80 mmHg, repeat in 2 months
- Use ACEI/CCB as appropriate.

LIPID MANAGEMENT

- Assess CVD risk annually including lipid profile
- Simvastatin first line.

ANTITHROMBOTIC THERAPY

- If over 50 years and BP < 145/90 mmHg
- If < 50 years and other significant CVD risk factors.

RENAL DISEASE

- Annual ACR – first-pass sample
- Annual creatinine and eGFR estimation
- Microalbuminuria if at least one ACR test is abnormal (> 2.5 mg/mmol for men or > 3.5 mg/mmol for women)
- Consider non-diabetic causes of renal disease
- Treat nephropathy with ACEI and aim for BP < 130/80 mmHg.

CHAPTER 7

CASE 13

INSTRUCTIONS TO CANDIDATES (CASE NOTES)

You have never met this patient before.

Name   Brian Dover

Age   48 years

Social and family history   Works as a carpenter, never smoked

Last entry in notes (2 weeks ago):

Home visit: Acute shortness of breath

                         Looks unwell

                         Respiratory rate 40/min

                         Pulse 120/min

                         Creps bibasally

                         Impression – acute LVF

                         Plan – refer to medics

Handwritten discharge letter from hospital:

Acute LVF, secondary to viral infection

Angio: NAD, echo: moderate left ventricular systolic dysfunction

Medications on discharge: Ramipril 5 mg od, GP, please check U&Es

                         Bisoprolol 5 mg od

                         Furosemide 20 mg od

Review, 2 months in clinic with repeat echo. Cardiac rehab.

CHAPTER 7

BRAINSTORM

INSTRUCTIONS TO ROLE PLAYER (PATIENT)

NOT TO BE SEEN BY THE CANDIDATE

Patient background:

You are Brian Dover, you are 48 years old.

You became suddenly short of breath 2 weeks ago and called for an urgent home visit.

You saw your usual GP, Dr Thakkar, he sent you into hospital.

You went to hospital for 5 days. You initially spent hours in the Emergency Department and were then admitted to the cardiac ward.

You had blood tests, radiographs and a specialist doctor scanned your heart. You also had a test, 'angio' something, to see if you have blocked arteries in your heart. Luckily that was normal.

The cardiologist said Dr Thakkar was spot on; that you had LVF and it was it was probably due to a virus.

Opening statement:

'Hi Doctor! I've come to get my pills!'

Freely divulged in response to open questions:

You don't get breathless when you lie flat in bed or when you walk to the local shops.

You haven't felt breathless at all since you left hospital.

You have no idea what LVF means.

You don't drink alcohol or smoke.

You were given 2 weeks supply of your pills and you have come to get some more.

Information divulged if asked specifically:

You don't know how long you have to take the medicines for.

You can't remember the drug doses, but you follow the instructions on the box.

You have had today's drugs, but don't have any left for tomorrow. You forgot to bring the boxes with you.

You are not quite sure what the drugs do.

You are worried what the future holds.

The hospital will be starting an exercise programme for you soon.

NOTES

DATA-GATHERING, TECHNICAL AND ASSESSMENT SKILLS

- The hospital discharge summary (see case notes) provides key information about his diagnosis, medication and follow-up.

- The main focus of this case is to ensure he understands his condition and its management (all this information is provided on the discharge summary).

- Does he know what happened to him?

- How is his breathing now?

- Does he have any symptoms of breathlessness – on exertion, at rest, orthopnoea, paroxysmal nocturnal dyspnoea?

- Is he getting side effects of drugs? (Look in the BNF if you can't remember although this may take up valuable time.)

- Check his pulse, blood pressure, auscultate his heart sounds and lung fields and check for pitting oedema, although the examiner may not allow you to examine him or the patient may refuse.

- Ask about what drugs he is on and if he knows what they are for.

- Does he know the drug doses and when to take them?

- Is he aware of how to get more drugs (repeat prescription system)?

- Does he know what the follow-up plans are – cardiac exercise programme and clinic follow-up?

CLINICAL MANAGEMENT SKILLS

- Inform him of what happened and why.

- Explain why he has been prescribed his drugs, what side effects to watch out for and how he can get more.

- Organise U&Es and explain why this is important. Explain that you will contact him if you are concerned about the results.

- Explain what he should do if he gets breathless.

- Prescribe the drugs he requires.

INTERPERSONAL SKILLS

- Getting the story from the patient, about what happened in hospital, may provide you with information about his understanding, health beliefs and concerns. Many people are fearful of heart disease.

- He has been through a frightening experience. To acknowledge how frightening this must have been for him may offer a channel for him to express his concerns.

- What are his ideas as to what happened? Did he think that he had a heart attack? Does he know what LVF means? What is his view when you use the word 'failure'?

- What are his expectations? Does he expect to achieve a full recovery?

- It would be difficult to offer an accurate prognosis, particularly without a formal hospital letter with the test results. It is reasonable to be honest and say that you don't have enough information at this stage; the hospital team will be able to provide more information on how he is doing once the second scan has been done in a few weeks' time.

- Offer hope rather than doom and gloom.

CHAPTER 7

- Suggest that he comes back in a few weeks, perhaps after he is seen in clinic, to see how he is doing; this may offer added support.

- Agree a plan of action between you and the patient that suits you both, eg follow-up, prescribing of drugs.

- It is important to summarise what you have said and check his understanding.

- Give him the opportunity to ask further questions that may be discussed at a later date, he may think of questions once he leaves the consulting room.

FURTHER READING

The European Society of Cardiology offer excellent documents on the treatment of cardiac failure and other cardiological conditions:

www.escardio.org

Key principles of management (LVSD) include:

- addressing co-morbidities and lifestyle

- education and monitoring

- uptitration of drugs

CHAPTER 7

BONUS CASE

IN THIS STATION ...

You are a new GP at the practice.

MATERIALS AND INSTRUCTIONS TO CANDIDATE (CASE NOTES)

Name	Henry Prince
Age	73
Address	4a Modbury Gardens, Chalk Farm, London NW5
Social and family history	Lives with wife, Cybil
Past medical history	Prostate cancer
Current medication	Diethylstilbestrol 1 mg two tablets od
	Aspirin 75 mg od
Letter from oncologist	See over page

London Cancer Unit NHS Trust

Switchboard: 0207 1110000

Department of Uro-oncology

Lead consultant: Professor R. Thakkar

Clinic date (last week)

Dear Dr

Re: Henry Prince

Age: 73

Address: 4a Modbury Gardens, Chalk Farm, London, NW5

Hosp no. 4964dwe6

Diagnosis: Transfusion-dependent metastatic prostate cancer

Treatment to date:

Bicalutamide

Diethylstilbestrol

Current PSA: 749

I reviewed Mr Prince in clinic without his wife this morning. His PSA was 84 three months ago but has now accelerated to 749. He is relatively symptom free. His current regimen is therefore now not effective. We had a frank discussion regarding the future and agreed that I will now hand over to palliative care. I'd be grateful if you arrange a referral to your local services.

Yours sincerely

Dr Hans Johansson

Associate specialist in oncology

BRAINSTORM

INSTRUCTIONS TO ROLE PLAYER (PATIENT OR CARER)

NOT TO BE SEEN BY THE CANDIDATE

You are Henry Prince, 73, a retired butcher.

You have prostate cancer, and were told to come to see the GP after seeing your specialist last week.

The doctor at the hospital said that you were palliative but you have no idea what that means.

Opening statement

'Hello doctor, I was asked to come to see you by my specialist. He said he'd be sending you a letter. Has it arrived?'

Freely divulged in response to open questions:

You have prostate cancer and medicines for it.

You don't feel too bad in yourself and don't experience much in the way of pain.

You have to have blood transfusions regularly. You are due to have another blood test in 2 weeks with the practice nurse.

Information divulged if asked specifically:

You don't take much notice of the PSA test; you know that it's related to prostate cancer but you don't really know what it means and what your readings are.

You wife understands it all but she couldn't make it here today, and she'd like the GP to call her later today if possible. You have signed a consent form for this. Her very elderly mother had a fall recently so your wife has had to spend a lot of time with her.

You don't understand how bad the cancer is.

You don't know what 'palliative' means; the doctor at the hospital used it many times.

You are shocked when you are told what palliative means, but deep down not surprised.

CHAPTER 7

You have questions about what will happen next: Will you be in pain?

You don't want to be managed in hospital and would like to die at home; you and your wife had already talked about this.

You would prefer to have cancer specialist nurses come to your home rather than come to the hospital.

You don't want to die in a hospice – but in all honesty you've never visited one.

You don't want to be resuscitated if your heart stops or you stop breathing.

NOTES

OVERALL AIM OF THE CASE

To break bad news to a patient that his or her cancer is terminal and to plan for the future accordingly.

DATA GATHERING, TECHNICAL AND ASSESSMENT SKILLS

- Establish the content of the consultation with the specialist.
- Establish the patient's symptoms to date.

CLINICAL MANAGEMENT SKILLS

- Putting plans in place for end-of-life care (the whole plan won't be established in 10 minutes but key principles can be agreed).
- Clear safety net and follow-up.
- Establish clear lines of communication.

- Consider written plans so that his wife can see.

- Referral to community palliative care teams.

- DNAR status.

- Plans submitted to the out-of-hours service.

INTERPERSONAL SKILLS

- Checking understanding.

- Sharing understanding.

- Explore and manage expectations.

- Agreeing a management plan together.

FACT FINDER

- Practical aspects of palliative care include (note that list not exhaustive):

- Establishing with the patient that he or she is now palliative.

- Understanding and managing patient's emotional state, wishes, ideas, concerns and expectations.

- Understanding patient's symptom complex and treating accordingly.

- Agreeing plans with the patient and carers, including DNAR status.

- Planning for future eventualities, including pain, nausea, agitation such as organising just-in-case medication, syringe driver.

- Planning disease-specific aspects, eg transfusions, pleural/ascitic taps.

- Ensuring that activities of daily living can be managed such as toileting, hydration.

- Ensuring that all parties are involved, including out-of-hours service.

Chapter 8
What next?

The MRCGP assesses the ability of a candidate to practise safely and effectively as an independent GP. The CSA aims to reflect everyday general practice cases rather than esoteric medicine, and preparation should be an ongoing process that occurs throughout GP training rather than a cramming exercise 2 weeks before the examination.

Between now and the examination try to treat every patient you see as a CSA case. Consult in a patient-centred way using recognised consultation models. Read up on the knowledge (eg guidelines) required to manage the problems that you come across during your consultations. Reflect on how you managed each case. How could you do better next time? What are your learning needs and how can you address these deficiencies?

The CSA is more than a test of consultation skills and disease management; it also tests examination skills. Unlike the MRCP, the clinical examinations required within the CSA are likely to focus on symptoms rather than systems. This being the case, in addition to considering the questions that you may need to ask, it is useful to practise examination of a patient with specific symptoms such as headaches, breathlessness, tiredness, and so on. You will also have to demonstrate that you can use medical equipment proficiently, such as peak flow meters, inhalers and obstetric calendars.

How can you know if you are consulting to the right standard? Make use of the consultation observational tool (COT). Organise joint surgeries with your trainer and the other GPs in your practice. This will demonstrate different techniques and consulting styles that you can adopt. Your trainer can also give you feedback and discuss ways in which you can improve your skills. Videoing your consultations and watching them back on your own, with peers or with your trainer, is a powerful tool. It will help you identify your strengths and more importantly, your weaknesses. You can also review the video consultations offered as free 'Online Extras' in conjunction with this book – see www.pastest.co.uk/online extras.

Role-playing cases, either on a course or with a colleague playing the patient and another observing, is invaluable and provides practice under 'examination conditions'.

The MRCGP should be a joy to prepare for. A planned approach, consistent application and dedication are required for success. Reflect on your

CHAPTER 8

learning needs, make use of the teachers around you and regularly visit the RCGP website.

Whichever way you approach the MRCGP, remember that your registrar year is supposed to be exciting, enlightening and, above all, enjoyable! Good luck!

INDEX